THE MEDICAL CLASSIC
OF THE YELLOW EMPEROR

Translated by
Zhu Ming

FOREIGN LANGUAGES PRESS · BEIJING

First Edition 2001
Second Printing 2005

Website:
http://www.flp.com.cn
Email Address:
Info@flp.com.cn
Sales@flp.com.cn

ISBN 7 – 119 – 02664 – X

ⓒ Foreign Languages Press, Beijing, China, 2001

Published by Foreign Languages Press
24 Baiwanzhuang Road, Beijing 100037, China
Distributed by China International Book Trading Corporation
35 Chegongzhuang Xilu, Beijing 100044, China
P. O. Box 399, Beijing, China

Printed in the People's Republic of China

Translator's Preface

With the rapid expansion of China's policy of openness, cultural exchange between the West and East is being greatly stimulated. Traditional Chinese medicine (TCM), as a distinctive element of East Asian civilization and one of the great medical traditions of the world, is attracting more and more interest. Awareness of acupuncture has spread widely in the Western society and TCM is also gaining recognition daily. Nowadays, highly advanced Western medicine is facing a kind of great Green Revolution that aims at producing more natural drugs and medical techniques without noxious side-effects. In contrast, millennia old TCM, which successfully united all scientific achievements in ancient times, has failed to absorb modern advanced technology in recent times and is confronted with a great challenge of modernization. Therefore, it is inevitable that ancient East Asian medical understanding will combine with modern Western medical knowledge to form a glorious whole, which our contemporaries and generations to come will appreciate as a great contribution to the cause of human health.

In Western countries scholars and physicians are engaged in systematic and comprehensive study of TCM and have made rapid progress both in theory and in practice. Naturally, many of these researchers into TCM are interested in knowing its earliest sources, which have been rendered mysterious and enticing by their inaccessibility. It is unfortunate, but there are three significant cultural and linguistic barriers to easy understanding: between English language and Chinese language, between standard Chinese and TCM technical terminology, and between modern TCM terminology and archaic medical Chinese. Few of the westerners who have tried to stride over the three wide gaps have been able to successfully approach this attractive and exotic medical field. Hence, more culture brokers are needed who are sufficiently proficient in TCM, on archaic medical Chinese and in English, so that more Western people can receive adequate information about the origins of TCM.

The Medical Classic of the Yellow Emperor (*Huang Di Nei Jing*), which is also translated by Ilza Veith as *The Yellow Emperor's Classic of Internal Medicine* (1966), is the oldest extant classic of TCM and the source of theory for this independent medical system. This book is written in the form of a dialogue in which the Yellow Emperor (the legendary first ancestor of the Chinese nation) discusses medicine with his ministers and some well-known doctors. No student of TCM in China could escape knowing about this text.

I made my decision to translate *The Medical Classic of the Yellow Emperor* into English after I became a doctor of TCM from the Hunan College of Traditional Chinese Medicine and had undertaken clinical practice of TCM for many years. Fearing that my translation would

I

do disservice to this great text, I proceeded meticulously in almost every step of my work, yet it was pushed forward slowly but surely by my faithfulness to, and enthusiasm for, the masterpiece.

The Original Version

A perfect version of the original text is a precondition for a satisfactorily translated product. I choose the textbook version of *The Medical Classic of the Yellow Emperor* as my original. It was edited by the Compiling and Checking Committee of Textbooks of State Universities and Colleges organized by the Ministry of Public Health of the People's Republic of China in 1982. The chief editor, Dr. Cheng Shide, is from Beijing TCM College. This textbook explains the original articles of *The Medical Classic of the Yellow Emperor* in a scientific, orderly and concise way. It is the unquestionably authoritative and consummate source. Annotations that quote explanatory notes of many famous ancient medical masters are presented as concisely as possible, while some necessary explanations are added.

Structure of This Book

The structure of this book is to present the translations of an original article, or a section of dialogue, from The *Medical Classic of the Yellow Emperor*, followed by annotations and commentaries. This stable structure is intended to constantly clarify the reader's understanding.

Sometimes, the original article and the annotations may convey a same concept in two different forms of expression. For example, the original article says, "Open the ghost gate and cleanse the clear *fu*-organ," while the annotation which follows says, "Diaphoresis and diuresis." The reason for the significant difference between the translation of the original article and the annotation is that, while words "diaphoresis and diuresis" present a readily recognizable gloss in Western medical terminology, a literal translation of the original text is closer to the expression accepted by practitioners of TCM in China and comes closer to reflecting the real meaning in the context of TCM conceptualization.

Most of the original articles of *The Medical Classic of the Yellow Emperor* are quite terse. Hence, in order to make the translations of each article as close as possible to the Chinese language source, the annotations making the concepts and sentences more complete and clearer, and the commentaries summing up the gist of the articles, are usually indispensable.

Style of Translation

Literal translation, freely conveying factual information, is dependable and is the technique of translation adopted here. Many books have been successfully translated word-for-word into English and published in order to introduce TCM to the world.

However, in an ordinary situation when an ancient classic of TCM is translated, dozens of experts from many fields take part in the work. First, professors of TCM interpret the book into current Chinese; then, professors of Western medicine, historians, linguists, anthropologists, etc., who have profound knowledge of English and Chinese, but not of TCM, translate this book into English. So, it is not difficult for us to imagine that errors due to different modes of thinking may occur. The different modes of thinking, different word usages, different styles and skills of translation, etc., may perplex readers. Western readers will frequently find inconsistencies in identifying concepts, just as if a man has five different names. The mistakes in disease names used in Western medicine will twist the facts fundamentally and confuse readers, especially among scholars of Western medicine. Thus, to translate verbatim is the best but hardest choice.

The principle of literal translation penetrates the entire proceeding of my work. Unavoidably, some words have to be added or deleted on some necessary occasions in order to offer a correct and full understanding. Some examples of literal translation are demonstrated as follows:

1. 邪 之 所 凑 , 其 气 必 虚 。

   Where evils converge, the *qi* must be deficient.

2. 正 气 存 内 , 邪 不 可 干 。

   The right *qi* exists inside; evils cannot make disturbance.

3. 壮 水 之 主 以 制 阳 光 。

   Strengthen the dominance of water to control the *yang* light.

4. 益 火 之 源 以 消 阴 翳 。

   Boost the source of fire to disperse the *yin* shadow.

5. 五 藏 者 , 所 以 藏 精 神 血 气 魂 魄 者 也 。

   The five *zang*-organs are what store the essence, spirit, blood, *qi*, *yang* soul, and *yin* soul.

6. 六 府 者 , 所 以 化 水 谷 而 行 津 液 者 也 。

   The six *fu*-organs are what transform water and grains and move the fluids.

Word Selection

All terms and concepts of TCM originate from the daily speech and activities of working people. It is easy to find their equivalents in English. English is based on people's shared experience in living, just as Chinese is. Therefore, English equivalents for terms in TCM can be determined. Generally speaking, any word that clearly conveys the true meaning of a Chinese term is acceptable. However, both Chinese and English have many synonyms, so a reliable and relatively stable system of terms is required. It is a matter for rejoicing that the system of terms is becoming more and more mature now in a universally recognized way after the efforts of many people from China and abroad. I have consulted many English books about TCM published in China and overseas. Of these, I tend to favor the work of the English enthusiast, Dr. Nigel Wiseman, who has made insightful and marvelous explorations in establishing the terminological system of TCM.

It is worthwhile to mention that it is not wise for us to try to equate the terms of TCM to those of Western medicine, inasmuch as it usually leads to conceptual mistakes. In general, the anatomical terms are compatible. We had better avoid using the terms of Western medicine in TCM, especially using disease names, which often risks committing fatal mistakes, because TCM and Western medicine research the same entity from utterly different angles.

I am confident that no expression in this book will seem too thorny when a foreign reader has grasped terms that frequently appear, such as *qi* (气), *yin* (阴), *yang* (阳), *zang*-organ(脏), *fu*-organ(腑), triple-warmer (三焦), nutritive *qi* (营), and defensive *qi* (卫). A lucid English version, which even a foreigner without any knowledge of TCM and Chinese culture can understand with ease, is what I have done my utmost to produce. As we all know, science has no borders. TCM, the great treasure, should belong to the world's people. I am sure the comprehensive exportation of TCM will bring a brighter future to the health cause of the human race.

Many sincere thanks are extended to Prof. Tong Yao and Prof. Yao Yong, working in Shanghai University of TCM now, for their instructive advice for modification. I also want to express my special gratitude to the international scholars of TCM, Prof. Stephen R. Smith of Wittenberg University in Springfield, Ohio, USA, Dr. Isabeau Volhardt, L. AC. of University of Washington, and Dr. Kim Taylor of University of Cambridge in England for their convincing and extensive revisions of my manuscript and their cordial encouragement. The English language is also corrected by Patti J. Tobin, Justin Sattin, Barry J. Grice, Volker Scheid, John Wm. Schiffeler, Gypsy Cole, Chao Yuan-Ling, Liu Xun, and Sun Ming, whose enthusiastic support for this project is admirable. The quality of the book would not have been improved without their generous help. Being impossible to be unassailable, this book eagerly awaits more criticism from all fields.

Zhu Ming

Huaihua, Hunan Province, China.

January 1, 2000.

Tel. 0086 – 0745 – 2350157

Email: zhuming6812@hotmail.com

CONTENTS

Introduction to
The Medical Classic of the Yellow Emperor

The Medical Classic of the Yellow Emperor is one of the earliest books found in the corpus of traditional Chinese medicine (TCM). It enunciates the systematic structure of the theoretical system of TCM and reflects the theoretical principles and academic thoughts associated with it. This theoretical system has formed the basis for development of TCM since its establishment. Nearly all academic thoughts of many well-known medical masters and medical schools appearing during the history of TCM have grown out of the theoretical system of *The Medical Classic of the Yellow Emperor*. Consequently, it is one of the basic theoretical curriculums of TCM today.

All medical theories come from practice and, in turn, direct practice. Throughout the millennia, the great contributions by TCM to ensure the well-being of Chinese people depended on the theoretical system of *The Medical Classic of the Yellow Emperor*. Therefore, it received lavish attention from medical practitioners throughout Chinese history and was venerated as an ancestral work of physicians, not to mention being a compulsory classical work in TCM.

Times of Compilation and Its Author

Many historians and physicians throughout Chinese history studied and verified that the major contents of *The Medical Classic of the Yellow Emperor* had appeared in the Warring States Period (475 BC — 221 BC). It had been added during the Qin Dynasty (221 BC — 206 BC) and Han Dynasty (206 BC — 220 AD), and had been compiled to the public at the early time of the Western Han Dynasty (206 BC — 24 AD).

The Yellow Emperor is the legendary first ancestor of the Chinese nation, and many Chinese people are proud of being regarded as his offspring. Many Chinese living in earlier times ascribed all their culture to him. This book was titled with his name in order to lead it to fame and authority. The academic divergence of thoughts in this book sufficiently indicates that it is neither a work of a single individual, nor medical achievement of a certain period or a local region, but rather the summarization of experiences of many medical practitioners over a long time.

Components of the Book

The currently universal version of *The Medical Classic of the Yellow Emperor* encompasses two parts, *The Plain Questions* and *The Divine Pivot*. Each part has eighty-one articles. Thus, the book is composed of one hundred and sixty-two articles.

Basic Academic Thoughts Found in the Theoretical System
of *The Medical Classic of the Yellow Emperor*

The compilation of *The Medical Classic of the Yellow Emperor* established the unique theoretical system of TCM, and formed the basis for the development of TCM. According to the development regularity of medicines and the inference from the theoretical contents of *The Medical Classic of the Yellow Emperor*, this distinct system is based on anatomical knowledge, and directed by ancient philosophical thoughts. It was produced after long observation of life's phenomena, and proved repeatedly through medical practice. It developed gradually to form from perceptual cognition to rational knowledge and from scraps to comprehensiveness. Therefore, the theoretical system described in this work is under the guidance of ancient plain materialist dialectics, combining with the regularity of human life's activities. This system also presents a lot of significant theoretical principles and academic thoughts. They are also ideological ways that we must master when we study *The Medical Classic of the Yellow Emperor*. This theoretical system has two typical features, i. e., plain materialist dialectics and integral idea that man and nature are mutually corresponding.

Plain Materialist Dialectics
  A. The "essential *qi*" is the source of the generation and formation of everything. The ancient Chinese philosophers regarded that the source of the cosmos was the essential *qi*. Everything in the world was produced by the essential *qi*, namely, original *qi*. The *qi* is an invisible materialistic element that forms everything. Of course, the "everything" also encompasses the human beings. Man is endowed with the essential *qi* from nature, and it is called *qi*, essential *qi*, vital *qi*, or original *qi*. The concept of *qi* permeated the medical field. Thus, the idea that everything consists of *qi* is inevitably shown in *The Medical Classic of the Yellow Emperor*. The *qi* is not only the basic material that forms the body, but also the dynamic power of the body. The life's activities of human beings are the manifestations of movements of the *qi*. Different combinations of the *qi* may generate different things. So, according to different places and different functioning of the *qi*, different names of *qi* are determined, such as true *qi*, ancestral *qi*, nutritive *qi*, defensive *qi*, liver *qi*,

spleen *qi*, heart *qi*, etc.

B. The materialism is highlighted. Prevailed the theories of *yin-yang* and the five elements in plain materialist dialectics, which were used to explain the changes of nature in the Spring and Autumn Period (770 BC — 476 BC) and Warring States Period (475 BC — 221 BC). It let more people become suspicious of the religious superstitions towards gods and ghosts. Life science was led to the realm of materialism.

C. The proposition that the life is antagonistic and united is prominent. Not only the body's structures but also life's activities are antagonistic and united, and too are man and nature. Everything has its two antagonistic and united sides, i.e., *yin* and *yang*. The antagonistic and united movements of the *yin* and *yang* push everything to develop forward incessantly, originating birth and death of everything.

D. Life is undergoing constant flux all the time. *The Medical Classic of the Yellow Emperor* regards the entity of nature, living things and diseases as not being motionless and still, but incessantly moving, developing and changing under the mutual actions of the *yin* and *yang*. Consequently, we should analyze and treat a disease with the idea of movement. This is the theoretical reference to syndrome identification and treatment determination in TCM.

The Integral Idea That Man and Nature Are Mutually Corresponding

Man and nature are mutually corresponding. This is a unique feature of TCM that differs from almost all other world medicines. TCM regards the physiological processes and pathological changes of human beings are closely related to nature. Many things involved are put into correspondences organically, such as the waxing and waning of the *yin* and *yang* of nature; the five elements that constitute the world, i.e., wood, fire, soil, metal and water; the running of the sun and moon and stars. The climatic changes of spring, summer, autumn and winter; the spring generation, summer growth, autumn harvest, and winter storage; the human functional system in which the five *zang*-organs are the chief body, and such things, are linked up as well. The occultness and the intrinsic links of both the universe and human beings are incredibly demonstrated.

Chapter Sorting

The Medical Classic of the Yellow Emperor was compiled over two thousand years ago. The language used in this book is archaic and laconic, and its expressions are gracious, far-reaching, and abstruse. The time when it was written is very distant. The book was copied again and again by hand. In ancient times people wrote on bamboo slips which were then tied together. Over the years the binding would sometimes fall apart and the slips would smudge or break. Therefore, pieces of the original text might become mixed up, in-

comprehensible or incomplete. This history gives us some difficulty in trying to study The Medical Classic of the Yellow Emperor.

In this book, all the contents of *The Medical Classic of the Yellow Emperor* are arranged in eight chapters, except for "acupuncture" and "five movements and six climatic *qi*." The eight chapters are respectively the *yin-yang* and the five elements, *zang*-organs and manifestations, channels and network-channels, pathogens and pathomechanisms, diseases and symptoms, diagnostic methods, therapeutic principles and methods, and health preservation.

Chapter One
Theory of *Yin-Yang* and
Theory of the Five Elements

The theory of *yin-yang* and the theory of the five elements are both based on the ideas of ancient Chinese philosophers who believed that everything in the universe originated from the *qi* (a metaphysical yet materialistic element that formed all matter). These theories are ascribed to the category of ancient Chinese philosophy, and are used to describe and explain all change of everything in the world.

The theory of *yin-yang* claims that everything in the physical world coexists in two opposite sides, and that the opposite and integral movements of the two halves provide the primitive impetus for all change and development. The *yin* and *yang* are used to describe these two closely related sides.

The theory of the five elements generally explains the interrelationships among moving things and their relatively stable state during movement. Its primary tenet is that the world is comprised of five elements: wood, fire, soil, metal and water. Each element can either promote or curb another. This phenomenon is referred to as either inter-promotion or inter-curb.

The theories of *yin-yang* and the five elements permeate the field of medical thought, forming the basis for the theoretical system of *The Medical Classic of the Yellow Emperor*, from which the theories of TCM originate. The theories are used to analyze and confirm the regularity of physiological processes and pathological changes in human beings, and they become important guidelines in the theories of TCM.

The following sections are extracted from the two parts of *The Medical Classic of the Yellow Emperor*, i.e., *The Plain Questions* and *The Divine Pivot*. These sections illustrate the rudimentary concepts of *yin-yang* and the five elements. They also include some principles relevant to physiology, pathology, diagnosis, and treatment.

1.1 Fifth Article

Great Topic on Correspondences and Manifestations of Yin and Yang ·
The Plain Questions (excerpt)

1.1.1 Original article

The Emperor[1] said:

The *yin* and *yang*[2] are the law of the heaven and earth, the rule of everything, the parents of variations, the root of life and death, and the locus of power of the universe. The root must be sought in treatment. So, accumulations of the *yang* constitute the heaven, and accumulations of the *yin* constitute the earth.[3] The *yin* is tranquil, and the *yang* is restless. As the *yang* is generated, the *yin* grows. As the *yang* is harsh, the *yin* is blockaded.[4] The *yang* produces the *qi*[5], and the *yin* produces forms.[6]

Extreme cold engenders heat, and extreme heat engenders cold.[7] The cold *qi* generates turbidity, and the hot *qi* generates clearness. If the clear *yang* is suppressed downward, it will cause diarrhea containing undigested foods.[8] If the turbid *yin* is carried upward, it will cause abdominal distention.[9] When the *yin* and *yang* are disordered, disease is induced.

Commentary

This section concisely describes the rudimentary concepts of *yin* and *yang*. It points out that everything in the world is constantly moving and changing, being born and vanishing. The root of every movement lies within the *yin* and *yang*. During the course of a movement, the two sides are not only mutually antagonistic, but also mutually dependent and facilitating. On certain occasions, they can transform each other. This proposition expresses that the theory of *yin-yang* incorporates the philosophical thoughts in materialist dialectics. The article also combines the theory of *yin-yang* with human physiology and pathology, and presents a fundamental principle in therapeutics that "the root must be sought in treatment."

Annotation

[1] The Emperor: The Yellow Emperor, who is regarded as the legendary first ancestor of the Chinese nation. *The Medical Classic of the Yellow Emperor* is a series of conversations between this emperor and his ministers and some well-known doctors, including Uncle Qi, Shao Yu, Lei Gong,

Bo Gao, Gui Yuqu, etc.

[2] The *yin* and *yang*: The attribute of *yin* or *yang* of a thing cannot be determined at random. A thing and its associated other thing, or the two sides of a thing, must be compared according to their intrinsic characteristics; then the attribute of *yin* or *yang* can be determined. Usually, the active, outward, ascending, warm, bright, functional, or hyper-functional pertain to the *yang*; the tranquil, inward, descending, cold, materialistic, or hypo-functional pertain to the *yin*. The *yin* and *yang* are not absolute, but relative.

[3] So, accumulations of the *yang* constitute the heaven, and accumulations of the *yin* constitute the earth: The *yang qi* is light and clear. The light things ascend. So, accumulations of the *yang* constitute the heaven. The *yin qi* is heavy and turbid. The heavy and turbid things descend. The *yin* coagulates, so accumulations of the *yin* constitute the earth.

[4] As the *yang* is generated, the *yin* grows. As the *yang* is harsh, the *yin* is blockaded: The *yin* and *yang* are mutually dependent. The former sentence suggests the normality of *yin* and *yang*; the next suggests the abnormality of *yin* and *yang*.

[5] The *qi*: The philosophers of ancient times regarded that the source of the cosmos was the "essential *qi*," and that everything in the world was produced by the essential *qi*. The *qi* is an invisible materialistic element that forms everything. Humans are endowed with the essential *qi* from nature, and it is called "*qi*," "essential *qi*," "vital *qi*," or "original *qi*." The concept of *qi* permeates the medical field. The *qi* is not only the basic material that forms the body, but also the dynamic power of the body.

[6] The *yang* produces the *qi*, and the *yin* produces forms: The *yang* is mobile and loose, so the *yang* produces the *qi*. The *yin* is quiet and coagulative, so the *yin* produces forms. The *qi* of everything is made of *yang*. The form of everything is made of *yin*. Therefore, the *qi* of the human body is called *yang qi*. The essence, blood and fluids are called true *yin*.

[7] Extreme cold engenders heat, and extreme heat engenders cold: The *yin* and *yang* can convert themselves mutually in certain situations. For example, a person suffering from a cold may get a fever. When the fever reaches its climax, the patient will shudder instead.

[8] If the clear *yang* is suppressed downward, it will cause diarrhea containing undigested foods: The clear *yang* dominates ascent. When it is weak at the lower part of the body and fails to ascend, diarrhea containing undigested foods ensues.

[9] If the turbid *yin* is carried upward, it will cause abdominal distention: The turbid *yin* dominates descent. When it is stagnant at the upper part of the body and fails to descend, abdominal distention results.

1.1.2 Original article

Hence, the clear *yang* makes the heaven, and the turbid *yin* makes the earth. The earthly qi^1 ascends to become clouds, and the heavenly qi^2 descends to become rain. Rain comes from the earthly *qi*, and clouds come from the heavenly *qi*.

So, the clear $yang^3$ gets out of the upper orifices[4], and the turbid yin^5 gets out of the lower orifices[6]. The clear $yang^7$ effuses the muscular striae[8], and the turbid yin^9 goes to the five *zang*-organs.[10] The clear $yang^{11}$ strengthens the four limbs, and the turbid yin^{12} flows to the six *fu*-organs[13].

Water is *yin*, and fire is *yang*. Smells of drugs are *yang*, and flavors of drugs are *yin*.

The flavors nourish the body form, and the *qi* nourishes the body form as well. The smells produce the body essence[14], and the *qi* produces the body essence as well.

The body essence is produced by the smells, and the body form is nourished by the flavors. The body essence is produced by the *qi*, and the body form is nourished by the *qi* as well.

The flavors impair the body form, and the smells impair the body essence[15]. The body essence transforms into qi^{16}, and the *qi* can also be harmed by the flavors.

Yin flavors get out of the lower orifices, and *yang* smells get out of the upper orifices. Thick flavors are *yin*, and thin flavors are *yang* within *yin*. Thick smells are *yang*, and thin smells are *yin* within $yang^{17}$. The thick flavor induces diarrhea, and the thin flavor promotes urination[18]. The thin smell produces sweating, and the thick smell produces heat[19]. The strong fire of a drug debilitates the *qi*, and a mild one strengthens the qi^{20}. The strong fire of a drug could devour the *qi*, but the *qi* could assimilate the mild fire of a drug. The strong fire could disperse the *qi*, but the mild fire could produce the *qi*.

Emanating and dissipating drugs with pungency and sweetness are *yang*. Emetic and laxative drugs with sourness and bitterness are *yin*. The *yin* being overwhelming, the *yang* becomes ill. The *yang* being overwhelming, the *yin* becomes ill. When the *yang* prevails, there is heat. When the *yin* prevails, there is cold. Double cold leads to heat, and double heat leads to cold. Cold damages the form, and heat damages the *qi*. The damaged *qi* causes pain, and the damaged form causes swelling[21]. Therefore, when the swelling follows the pain, the damaged *qi* harms the form. When the pain follows the swelling, the damaged form harms the *qi*.

Overwhelming wind causes stirring. Overwhelming heat causes swelling. Overwhelming dryness causes desiccation. Overwhelming cold causes edema. Overwhelming dampness causes laxation.

The heaven has the four seasons and the five elements that cause the cycle of generation, growth, reaping and storage; and cold, summer heat, dryness, dampness and wind are produced. A man has five *zang*-organs to generate the *qi* of the five *zang*-organs, so that joy, anger, sorrow, melancholy and fear are produced. Hence, excessive joy and anger injure the *qi*, and cold and summer heat injure the body form[22].

Tempestuous anger impairs the *yin*, and frantic joy impairs the *yang*[23]. The reverse *qi* moves upward — the full pulse loses its normal shape at that point. When joy and anger are intemperate, and cold and summer heat are excessive, one's life will not be secure. So, double *yin* must lead to *yang*, and double *yang* must lead to *yin*.

Hence the saying: Impaired by cold in winter, one must get a pyretic disease in spring[24]; impaired by wind in spring, one must get diarrhea containing undigested foods in summer[25]; spoiled by summer heat in summer, one must be afflicted with malaria in autumn[26]; spoiled by dampness in autumn, one must be afflicted with cough in winter[27].

Commentary

This article mainly discusses the heaven and earth, water and fire, clearness and turbidity, smell and flavor, physiology and pathology, etc. Upon these, the rudimentary contents of the theory of *yin-yang* are elucidated, such as the attributes of *yin* and *yang*, mutual dependence, descent, ascent, and mutual conversion.

The feature that the clear *yang qi* runs upward and outward and that the turbid *yin qi* runs downward and inward, provided many theoretical references to therapeutic methods in later eras. For example, the remedy of invigorating and lifting the *qi* is applied to treat deafness and blindness. The remedy of diffusing the lung *qi* and resolving the exterior is adopted to treat exterior syndrome, i.e., a cold. The remedy of warming the *yang* is used to treat cold arms and feet. The remedy of offensive defecation is used to treat food accumulation in the stomach and intestines. The remedy of excreting urine and expelling water is used to heal edema, and so on. These remedies are all enlightened by this theory.

As for the interrelationships of conversion among flavor, form, *qi* and blood, these are mainly used to explain a series of food metabolizing processes. Yet, the reasons never go beyond the ideas that the *yang* ascends and the *yin* descends, that the *yang* produces the *qi* and the *yin* produces forms, and that the *yang* is rooted in the *yin* and the *yin* is rooted in the *yang*.

Every drug has its own smell and flavor. Because of different smells and flavors, every drug possesses its own unique property. The smells and flavors have differences in thickness and thinness, have distinctions of heat, cold, warmth and coolness, and have specialties of sourness, bitterness, sweetness, saltiness, acridness and insipidness. What we notice in this article is from the angle of *yin* and *yang*. The properties of smells and flavors of drugs are given a general summarization here. This not only offers the theoretical basis of Chinese materia medica, but also forms the basis for development and classification of Chinese medicines.

The following table should be helpful in understanding the *yin* and *yang*:

Classification Table of *Yin* and *Yang*

yin	*yang*
water	fire
night	day
earth	heaven
cold	hot
autumn, winter	spring, summer
dark	bright
turbid	clear
still	mobile
bottom	top
inward	outward
chest	back
flavor	smell
blood, fluids	vital *qi*
lower orifices	upper orifices
weak	strong
visible	invisible
materialistic	spirited (functional)
zang-organs	*fu*-organs
female	male
black	white (red)
right side	left side
astringent	emanating

To facilitate the study of the following passages, please scan the table below:

Systematic Correspondence Table of
Nature — *Yin-Yang* — Man

nature	five directions	east	south	center	west	north
nature	five seasons	spring	summer	late summer	autumn	winter
nature	five airs	wind	heat	dampness	dryness	cold
nature	five actions	generation	growth	bloom	harvest	storage
nature	five elements	wood	fire	soil	metal	water
yin-yang	five attributes	lesser — *yang*	greater — *yang*	arriving — *yin*	lesser — *yin*	greater — *yin*
man	five *zang*-organs	liver	heart	spleen	lungs	kidneys
man	five *fu*-organs	gallbladder	small intestine	stomach	large intestine	bladder
man	five tissues	sinews	vessels	muscles	skin	bones
man	five sense organs	eyes	tongue	mouth	nose	ears
man	five manifested parts of bloom	nails	face	lips	body hair	hair
man	five colors	blue	red	yellow	white	black
man	five musical scales	*do*	*re*	*mi*	*so*	*la*
man	five sounds	shouting	laughing	singing	crying	moaning
man	five flavors	sour	bitter	sweet	acrid	salty
man	five emotions	anger	joy	thought	sorrow	fear
man	five odors	rammish	burned	fragrant	fishy	rancid

Annotation

[1] The earthly *qi*: in this context, vapor.

[2] The heavenly *qi*: in this context, vapor condensed by cold.

[3] The clear *yang*: in this context, tears, saliva, exhaled air, nasal mucus, etc.

[4] The upper orifices: the ears, eyes, nose and mouth.

[5] The turbid *yin*: in this context, stool, urine, menstruation, etc.

[6] The lower orifices: the anus, urethra and vagina.

[7] The clear *yang*: in this context, the defensive *qi* that is the turbid part of the essential *qi* from water and grains. The defensive *qi* pertains to the *yang* and protects the body surface like a fence. It is also called defensive *yang*.

[8] The muscular striae: spaces or interstices between the skin and muscles.

[9] The turbid *yin*: in this context, the essence, blood, or fluids.

[10] The five *zang*-organs: These are the five solid viscera, including the liver, heart, spleen, lungs and kidneys.

[11] The clear *yang*: in this context, the essential *qi* produced from water and grains.

[12] The turbid *yin*: in this context, metabolic waste material from water and grains.

[13] The six *fu*-organs: These are the six hollow organs, including the gallbladder, small intestine, stomach, large intestine, bladder and triple-warmer (water network).

[14] The body essence: Sperm or ovum.

[15] The flavors impair the body form, and the smells impair the body essence: If the flavor of a drug is too excessive, it will damage the body form. If the smell of a drug is too excessive, it will damage the body essence.

[16] The body essence transforms into *qi*: The *qi* could nourish the body essence, while the body essence could transform into *qi*. That is to say, the *qi* and body essence could transform mutually.

[17] Thick flavors are *yin*, and thin flavors are *yang* within *yin*. Thick smells are *yang*, and thin smells are *yin* within *yang*: This statement manifests that the *yin* and *yang* are endlessly dividable.

[18] The thick flavor induces diarrhea, and the thin flavor promotes urination: For example, rhubarb rhizome, which has the thickest flavor and severe cold, could quicken defecation of stool. Manshurian aristolochia stem with an insipid flavor could stimulate urination.

[19] The thin smell produces sweating, and the thick smell produces heat: For example, ephedra, which has slight acridness, warmth and a thin smell, plays a diaphoretic role. Lateral root of aconite, which has great acidity, heat and a thick smell, could create a feeling of heat.

[20] The strong fire of a drug debilitates the *qi*, and a mild one strengthens the *qi*: For example, monkshood is of great acridity and heat, and one's *qi* cannot override the strong fire, so the *qi* is made debilitated; ginseng, which has slight warmth, is a good tonic drug.

[21] The damaged *qi* causes pain, and the damaged form causes swelling: The *qi* likes smoothness. When the *qi* is impaired, stagnation will appear. The stagnation induces pain. When the form is damaged, the *qi* and blood linger and accumulate there, so swelling ensues.

[22] Hence, excessive joy and anger injure the *qi*, and cold and summer heat injure the body form: The joy and anger here represent the five emotions. The cold and summer heat here represent the six exogenous evils. The five emotions engender from within, so they first injure the *qi*. The six evils attack from outside, so they first injure the body form.

[23]Tempestuous anger impairs the *yin*, and frantic joy impairs the *yang* : The blood is *yin*. The liver stores the blood. Tempestuous angers damage the liver and blood, i.e., the *yin*. Frantic joy may frustrate the heart *yang*.

[24]Impaired by cold in winter, one must get a pyretic disease in spring: This is what is known as "latency of evil." If one is hit by cold evil in the winter, and if he does not get ill instantly, the cold evil becomes latent in the body. When the spring comes, the internal cold evil intermingles with the exogenous *yang* evils, and a pyretic disease occurs. We can easily see that the cold evil is *yin* and a pyretic disease is *yang*. It proves that double *yin* must lead to *yang*.

[25]Impaired by wind in spring, one must get diarrhea containing undigested foods in summer: This is also latency of evil. If one is hit by wind in the spring, and if he does not get ill at once, the evil becomes latent in the body. When the summer comes, the spleen is on duty. Because wind pertains to wood, so the wood curbs the soil. Diarrhea containing undigested foods appears. Wind is *yang* and diarrhea pertains to *yin*. This condition proves that double *yang* must lead to *yin*.

[26]Spoiled by summer heat in summer, one must be afflicted with malaria in autumn: If summer heat cannot be dissipated, it stays inside the body. When the autumn comes, the body surface is wrapped by coolness. So, the fire fights against the metal, and the cold combats with the heat. Malaria is induced.

[27]Spoiled by dampness in autumn, one must be afflicted with cough in winter: If one is hit by dampness in the autumn, and if he does not get ill at once, the damp evil becomes latent. When the winter comes, the dampness gradually turns into heat. The outside is chilly and the inside is hot. The disease is transmitted to the lungs, so a cough appears. Dampness is *yin* and cough with inflammation pertains to *yang*. Double *yin* must lead to *yang*.

1.1.3 Original article

The Emperor said: "I was told that the distantly ancient sages had discussed and researched into the body structures and that they had arrayed and distinguished the *zang-fu* organs. They had sought for links among the channels and defined the six correspondences in terms of the routes of the twelve main channels.[1] All acupuncture points had been named. All muscles and bones had been defined. The floating network-channels at the separate parts of the superficies had been listed. The changes of the four seasons and *yin* and *yang* all had regularity. Do you believe this?"

Uncle Qi answered: "The east produces wind. The wind promotes the wood *qi*. The wood *qi* generates sour flavor. The sour flavor nourishes the liver. The liver governs the sinews. The liver promotes the heart and dominates the eyes.

"To the heaven, the changes of *yin* and *yang* are mysterious and abstruse. To men, life's activities are never outside the realm of these changes. To the earth, the changes generate everything. Just because of these changes, the five flavors are generated. Man's wisdom is promoted, and the mystical nature of the universe is produced.

"The wind in the heaven, wood in the earth, sinews in the body, liver in the *zang*-organs, blue in colors, *jiao* (i.e., *do*) in musical scales,[2] shout in sounds, cramp in diseases, eyes in the orifices, sourness in flavors, and anger in emotions are all corresponding. Anger damages the liver, but sorrow can overcome anger.[3] Wind harms the sinews, but dryness can overcome wind.[4] Sourness impairs the sinews, but acridness can overcome sourness.[5]

"The south produces heat. The heat promotes the fire *qi*. The fire *qi* generates bitter flavor. The bitter flavor nourishes the heart. The heart governs the blood. The heart promotes the spleen, and dominates the tongue. The heat in the heaven, fire in the earth, vessels in the body, heart in the *zang*-organs, red in colors, *zhi* (*re*) in musical scales, laugh in sounds, melancholy in diseases, tongue in the orifices, bitterness in flavors, and joy in emotions are all corresponding. Joy damages the heart, but fear can overcome joy. Heat harms the *qi*, but cold can overcome heat. Bitterness impairs the *qi*, but saltiness can overcome bitterness.

"The center produces dampness. The dampness promotes the soil *qi*. The soil *qi* generates sweet flavor. The sweet flavor nourishes the spleen. The spleen governs the muscles. The spleen promotes the lungs, and dominates the mouth. The dampness in the heaven, soil in the earth, muscles in the body, spleen in the *zang*-organs, yellow in colors, *gong* (*mi*) in musical scales, singing in sounds, hiccup in diseases, mouth in the orifices, sweetness in flavors, and thought in emotions are all corresponding.

"Thought damages the spleen, but anger can overcome thought. Dampness harms the muscles, but wind can overcome dampness. Sweetness impairs the muscles, but sourness can overcome sweetness.

"The west produces dryness. The dryness promotes the metal *qi*. The metal *qi* generates acrid flavor. The acrid flavor nourishes the lungs. The lungs govern the skin and body hair[6]. The lungs promote the kidneys, and dominate the nose. The dryness in the heaven, metal in the earth, skin and body hair in the body, lungs in the *zang*-organs, white in colors, *shang* (*so*) in musical scales, cry in sounds, cough in diseases, nose in the orifices, acridness in flavors, and sorrow in emotions are all corresponding. Sorrow damages the lungs, but joy can overcome sorrow. Dryness harms the skin and body hair, but heat can overcome dryness. Acridness impairs the skin and body hair, but bitterness can overcome acridness.

"The north produces cold. The cold promotes the water *qi*. The water *qi* generates salty flavor. The salty flavor nourishes the kidneys. The kidneys govern the marrow. The kidneys promote the liver, and dominate the ears. The cold in the heaven, water in the earth, bones in the body, kidneys in the *zang*-organs, black in colors, *yu* (*la*) in musical scales, moan in sounds, shudder in diseases, ears in the orifices, saltiness in flavors, and fear in emotions are all corresponding. Fear damages the kidneys, but thought can overcome fear. Cold harms the blood, but dryness can overcome cold. Saltiness impairs the blood, but sweetness can overcome saltiness.

"Hence the saying: Everything exists between the heaven and earth. The *yin* and *yang* decide the *qi*, blood, male and female. The left and right are the ways of the *yin* and *yang*.[7] Water and fire are the verification of the *yin* and *yang*. The *yin* and *yang* are the root of everything. So it is said that: The *yin* that stays inside is the defender of the *yang*; the *yang* that stays outside goes errands for the *yin*.[8]"

Commentary

The foregoing article uses the theories of *yin-yang* and the five elements to connect matters in nature with matters relating to man's actual viscera and tissues. It roughly chalks out the outline of systematic framework of the "four seasons, five *zang*-organs and *yin-yang*." The systematic comparison of multiple characteristics of the "four seasons, five *zang*-organs and *yin-yang*" is the cardinal content of the theory of *zang*-organs and manifestations that will be explained in the following chapter. This content demonstrates the relationships of inter-promotion and inter-curb among the five *zang*-organs and the close tie between man and nature. The integral idea of the theoretical system of *The Medical Classic of the Yellow Emperor* comes through prominently here.

After lengthy observation of shows and manifestations of the *zang*-organs, ancient medical masters and doctors summarized that the human body adapts to natural changes easily. By their work, they came to understand the systematic division of the functional activities of the five *zang*-organs. The theory of *zang*-organs and manifestations points out that life's activities are affected by external factors, such as natural circumstances, etc. Of course, these factors are only the external causes of life's activities. There must be a kind of corresponding mechanism inside the body. This discussion proposes a new way for us to collect and collate TCM research in a modern, scientific way.

Annotation

[1] The six correspondences in terms of the routes of the twelve main channels: The foot greater-*yin* spleen channel and foot bright-*yang* stomach channel are a couple. The foot cold-*yin* liver channel and foot lesser-*yang* gallbladder channel are a correspondence. The foot lesser-*yin* kidney channel and foot greater-*yang* bladder channel are a couple. The hand greater-*yin* lung channel and hand bright-*yang* large-intestine channel are a correspondence. The hand cold-*yin* pericardium channel and hand lesser-yang triple-warmer channel are a correspondence. The hand lesser-*yin* heart channel and hand greater-*yang* small-intestine channel are a couple.

[2] *Jiao* (i.e., *do*) in musical scales: The ancient Chinese musical scales — *jiao*, *zhi*,

gong, *shang* and *yu* are roughly equivalent to the five modern musical scales — 1 (*do*), 2 (*re*), 3 (*mi*), 5 (*so*) and 6 (*la*). Different musical sounds have direct effects on the *zang-fu* organs. For example, music with melodious tones and lively rhythms could make people joyous and relaxed and also strengthen normal physiological functions of the *zang-fu* organs to help people live longer. On the other hand, music with an excessively strong beat or dispirited tones could make people feel unpleasant and harm the viscera.

[3] Anger damages the liver, but sorrow can overcome anger: As to anger, joy, thought, sorrow and fear: anger curbs thought, joy curbs sorrow, thought curbs fear, sorrow curbs anger, and fear curbs joy.

[4] Wind harms the sinews, but dryness can overcome wind: As to wind, heat, dampness, dryness and cold: wind curbs dampness, heat curbs dryness, dampness curbs cold, dryness curbs wind, and cold curbs heat.

[5] Sourness impairs the sinews, but acridness can overcome sourness: As to sourness, bitterness, sweetness, acridness and saltiness: sourness curbs sweetness, bitterness curbs acridness, sweetness curbs saltiness, acridness curbs sourness, and saltiness curbs bitterness.

[6] Body hair: The fine hair covering the entire body, excluding the hair of the head.

[7] The left and right are the ways of the *yin* and *yang*: The left is *yang* and the right is *yin*.

[8] The *yin* that stays inside is the defender of the *yang*; the *yang* that stays outside goes errands for the *yin*: The *yin* and *yang* depend upon and transform each other.

1.1.4 Original article

The Emperor asked: "What about unbalanced *yin* and *yang*? "

Uncle Qi answered: "Overwhelming *yang* causes fever, closed muscular striae, rough gasping, bending back and forth, absence of sweat, a hot body, dry teeth, a stuffy and depressive chest, and a full abdomen. It is fatal. The patient can bear winter, but cannot tolerate summer. The overwhelming *yin* causes a cold body, sweating, frequent shivers from cold, cold limbs, and a full abdomen. It is too deadly. The patient can bear summer, but cannot tolerate winter. The unbalanced *yin* and *yang* bring about different symptoms."

The Emperor asked: "How to regulate the *yin* and *yang*?"

Uncle Qi answered: "Unless sexual austerity is used to help to balance the *yin* and *yang*, premature senility may come. At forty, the kidney *qi* is reduced by half, and the constitution becomes debilitated. At fifty, the body becomes cumbersome, and the hearing and sight are no longer clear. At sixty, impotence arises. The *qi* becomes greatly enfeebled, and the nine orifices become impeded. The *yang qi* is vacuous at the lower part of the body, and the *yin qi* is replete at the upper part of the body, so the nose is runny and the eyes are watery. [1]

"So we say: One who knows this will be strong; one who does not will be senile. The two kinds of men enjoy different ages. The intelligent one will agree with it, but the stupid one will disagree. The stupid has deficient kidney *qi*, but the intelligent has a surplus of it. The surplus kidney *qi* makes the ears and eyes clear, the body sinewy and agile, the aged vigorous, and the young stronger. Therefore, the sages lead placid, austere and optimistic lives, and they can live to a great age. This is how the sages build their bodies."

The *yang qi* is deficient at the northwest. Hence, the northwest is *yin*, and left ear and eye are clearer than the right ear and eye. The *yin* is deficient at the southeast. Thus, the southeast is *yang*, and the right arm and leg are stronger than the left arm and leg.

The Emperor asked: "Why is this so?"

Uncle Qi answered: "The east is *yang*. The essence of *yang* stays at the upper part of the body. Therefore, the upper part is replete and the lower

part is deficient. The left eye and ear are clearer, and the use of the left arm
and leg are not convenient. The west is *yin*. The essence of *yin* stays at the
lower part of the body. Therefore, the lower part is replete and the upper part
is deficient. The right ear and eye are not clear, and the use of the right arm
and leg are convenient. When they are attacked by exogenous evils, the upper part of the right side and the lower part of the left side will be affected
more seriously. Because the *yin* and *yang* of the heaven and earth cannot remain unassailable, evils dwell in the weak parts.

"So, the heaven has essential *qi*, and the earth has forms.[2] The heaven
has eight solar terms, and the earth has five directions.[3] Thus, the heaven
and earth are eligible to be parents of everything. The clear *yang* rises to the
heaven, and the turbid *yin* descends to the earth. Thus, activities of the
heaven and earth are subject to the rule of *yin* and *yang*. So, generation,
growth, reaping and storage cycle endlessly.

"Only sages respond to the heaven to nurture their heads, respond to the
earth to nurture their legs, and respond to human matters to nurture the five
zang-organs. The heavenly *qi* flows to the lungs. The earthly *qi* runs to the
throat. The wind *qi* goes to the liver. The thunder *qi* gets to the heart. The
grain *qi* flows to the spleen. The rain *qi* rushes to the kidneys. The six channels are the rivers of the body. The intestines and stomach are the sea of water
and grains. The nine orifices are where waters rush out. To analogize men
and nature: Sweat could be named Rain, gasp could be named Speedy Wind,
and rage could be named Thunder. The reverse *qi* of a man is similar to the
heavenly *qi* not descending and the earthly *qi* not ascending. So, if health
care does not observe the rules of the heaven and earth, mishaps will certainly
occur."

Commentary

This article elaborates on the waxing and waning of *yin* and *yang*, the course of
man's growth, functional differences between the left and right, and certain physiological
phenomena. It expounds why and how mankind should abide by the rules of nature. It further stresses the academic principle that man and nature are correspondingly and reciprocally related.

Annotation

[1] The *yang qi* is vacuous at the lower part of the body, and the *yin qi* is replete at the upper part of the body, so the nose is runny and the eyes are watery: The *yang qi* is vacuous and fails to transform water.

[2] The heaven has essential *qi*, and the earth has forms: The ancient people regarded that the sun was the ancestor of the essential *qi* of *yang*, and the moon was the ancestor of the essential *qi* of *yin*. Jupiter (or Wood Star), Mars (or Fire Star), Saturn (or Soil Star), Venus (or Metal Star), and Mercury (or Water Star) are the ancestors of the essential *qi* of wood, fire, soil, metal and water. The essential *qi* of the five elements descended to the earth, and then the forms of all things were made.

[3] The heaven has eight solar terms, and the earth has five directions: There are twelve solar terms in all. But here, the eight solar terms refer to the Beginning of Spring, Beginning of Summer, Beginning of Autumn, Beginning of Winter, Spring Equinox, Autumn Equinox, Summer Solstice and Winter Solstice. The five directions are the east, south, west, north and center.

1.1.5 Original article

"Evils come like swift winds and rain, so experienced doctors first treat the skin and body hair, then the muscles, then the sinews and vessels, then the six *fu*-organs, and last the five *zang*-organs. In treating the five *zang*-organs, the patient is half alive and half dead. Thus, evils of the heaven usually poison the five *zang*-organs. Cold and heat of water and grains usually poison the six *fu*-organs. The dampness of the earth often poisons the skin, muscles, sinews and vessels.

"So, an adept doctor of acupuncture always needles the *yang* part when the *yin* part is ill,[1] and needles the *yin* part when the *yang* part is ill. He adjusts the right to treat the left, and adjusts the left to treat the right.[2] He must know himself to know his patients, and must know the exterior to know the interior. Detecting a surplus pulse, he must know a deficient one. Seeing the appearance of a disease, he foretells its development. This ensures no delay in treatment.

"Observing colors and taking the pulse, a doctor versed in diagnosis first distinguishes the *yin* from *yang*. The doctor observes the facial clearness and turbidity and separates the color parts of the face. By observing gasps and listening to sounds, he knows what the patient is suffering from. Taking the pulse, he identifies the disease. By pressing the *chi* and *cun* parts[3] at the wrist and noticing the floating, sinking, slippery, or uneven pulse, the doctor understands why the disease has occurred. Thus, correct diagnostic method leads to a perfect treatment."

Commentary

This article explicates the methods of diagnosis and treatment, which are required to follow the rules of *yin* and *yang*. The intruding sequence of exogenous evils from the exterior to the interior not only demonstrates the idea of pre-protection in the early therapeutic phase in TCM, but also plays a large role in diagnosis and treatment of exopathic diseases. The rules "needle the *yang* part when the *yin* part is ill, needle the *yin* part when the *yang* part is ill, adjust the right to treat the left, and adjust the left to treat the right," are still widely used today. They are a very important part in acupuncture treatment. Particularly, in pulse-taking and color-observation, one should distinguish the *yin* from *yang*, as this is the principle of diagnosis.

Annotation

[1] Needles the *yang* part when the *yin* part is ill: The *yin* part refers to the five *zang*-organs, *yin* channels, chest, abdomen, lower part of the body, etc. The *yang* part refers to the six *fu*-organs, *yang* channels, back, upper part of the body, etc.

[2] Adjusts the right to treat the left, and adjusts the left to treat the right: The *qi*, blood, *yin* and *yang* are linked in an up-and-down arrangement.

[3] Pressing the *chi* and *cun* parts: The wrist pulse is divided into three parts, called *cun* part, *guan* part and *chi* part, from the distal end to the proximal end of the arm.

1.2   Fourth Article

Discussion of the True Speeches of the Golden Cabinet·
The Plain Questions

1.2.1   Original article

The Emperor asked: "What are the eight winds of the heaven[1] and the five winds of the channels?[2]"

Uncle Qi answered: "The evils of the eight winds trespass through the channels to touch the five *zang*-organs and induce disease. What are known as 'seasonal curbs' are that spring curbs late summer; late summer curbs winter; winter curbs summer; summer curbs autumn; autumn curbs spring.[3]

"The east-wind evil emerges in spring and attacks the liver through the points of the head. The south-wind evil emerges in summer and attacks the heart through the points of the breast and the sides of the ribs. The west-wind evil emerges in autumn and attacks the lungs through the points of the shoulders and back. The north-wind evil emerges in winter and attacks the kidneys through the points of the loins and hips. The central evil pertains to soil and attacks the spleen through the points of the spine. That is to say, spring evils attack the head, summer evils attack the heart, autumn evils attack the shoulders and back, and winter evils attack the loins, hips and limbs.

"Thus, runny nose, nasal congestion and nosebleed often occur in spring. Diseases of the breast and rib-sides often occur in summer. Excessive diarrhea and coldabdomen usually arise in late summer. Wind malaria[4] usually occurs in autumn. Numb and cold limbs ordinarily appear in winter.

"If the patient uses appropriate massage and exercise, he will not have a runny nose, nasal congestion, nosebleed, or other neck disease in spring, and will not have disease of the breast and rib-sides in summer. He will not have excessive diarrhea and cold abdomen in late summer, will not have wind malaria in autumn, and will not have numb and cold limbs in winter. The essence of the kidneys is the root of the body. So a man who stores enough kidney essence in winter will not get a pyretic disease in spring. However, a man who does not sweat in summer will get wind malaria in autumn. This is an ordinary diagnostic principle."

Commentary

This article describes the common law of the action of the eight wind evils on the five *zang*-organs in the four seasons, and deals with the conditions of disordered places in different seasons. Further, two questions are especially discussed: First, that the care of the *qi* of *zang*-organs, especially the kidney *qi*, is critical to prevent from occurrence of disease in the four seasons. Second, that "if a man does not store enough kidney essence in winter, he will get a pyretic disease in spring." This idea was the theoretical basis for the theory of latent evil leading to febrile diseases in later periods of time.

Annotation

[1] The eight winds of the heaven: The eight winds in nature, respectively from the east, south, west, north, northwest, northeast, southwest and southeast. If the eight winds arrive in seasons, they are normal climates; otherwise they are evils that can make people ill.

[2] The five winds of the channels: They are also the five winds of the five *zang*-organs — the liver wind, heart wind, spleen wind, lung wind and kidney wind. All these are induced by the exogenous eight winds.

[3] What are known as "seasonal curbs" are that spring curbs late summer; late summer curbs winter; winter curbs summer; summer curbs autumn; autumn curbs spring: If a season experiences the kind of weather that belongs to its curbing season, it is abnormal, and diseases will occur. For example, if the climate of summer appears in autumn, or the climate of winter appears in summer, this is abnormal, and diseases will occur.

[4] Wind malaria: A kind of malaria. If a man does not sweat in the summer, the summer heat evil may lie latent in the body. When the harsh autumn comes, the heat evil inside the body conflicts with the external cold metal, and wind malaria appears.

1.2.2 Original article

"Hence the saying: There is *yang* within *yin*, and there is *yin* within *yang*. From dawn to midday is the *yang* of a day, and also the *yang* within *yang*. From midday to dusk is the *yang* of a day, and also the *yin* within *yang*. From dusk to midnight is the *yin* of a day, and also the *yin* within *yin*. From midnight to dawn is the *yin* of a day, and also the *yang* within *yin*. Man's nature corresponds to this as well.

"Regarding the *yin* and *yang* of a man, the exterior is *yang*, and the interior is *yin*. Regarding the *yin* and *yang* of the body, the back is *yang*, and the abdomen is *yin*. Regarding the *zang-fu* organs, the *zang*-organs are *yin*, and the *fu*-organs are *yang*. The five *zang*-organs (liver, heart, spleen, lungs and kidneys) are *yin*. The six *fu*-organs (the gallbladder, small intestine, stomach, large intestine, bladder and triple-warmer[1]) are *yang*.

"What about the *yin* within *yang* and the *yang* within *yin*? The *yin* (kidneys) get ill in winter, and the *yang* (heart) gets ill in summer. The *yin* (liver) gets ill in spring, and the *yang* (lungs) get ill in autumn. Acupuncture should be used in terms of the disordered places. The back is *yang*. The heart is the *yang* within *yang*, and the lungs are the *yin* within *yang*. The abdomen is *yin*. The kidneys are the *yin* within *yin*, and the liver is the *yang* within *yin*. In addition, the spleen is the beginning part of the *yin*.[2] The correspondences of the *yin* and *yang*, exterior and interior, inside and outside, and the *zang*-organs and *fu*-organs of man respond to the *yin* and *yang* of nature."

Commentary

The *yin* and *yang* of nature correspond to the *yin* and *yang* of man. This article analyzes the attributes of *yin* and *yang* of the body structures concretely. This is one of basic principles in the application of the theory of *yin-yang* to the human body. It explains the divisibility and relativity of the *yin* and *yang* of the body. Especially important are the attributes of *yin* and *yang* of the five *zang*-organs to physiology, pathology, and "syndrome identification and treatment determination" of the five *zang*-organs.

Annotation

[1] Triple-warmer: In TCM, the metabolic system of water is called the "triple-warmer." In an

ordinary situation, a body trunk is divided into three parts, i.e., the upper part, middle part, and lower part. These parts are respectively called "upper-warmer," "middle-warmer," and "lower-warmer." The triple-warmer is not a definite organ in modern anatomy. The triple-warmer is the water network of the body, and so it dominates the metabolism of body water and fluids. It is called a "warmer" because it warms and transforms water.

[2] The spleen is the beginning part of the *yin*: The spleen stays inside the abdomen. It corresponds to late summer outside, which connects with spring-summer and autumn-winter. It is from the *yang* to *yin*. So the spleen is the beginning part of the *yin*.

1.2.3 Original article

The Emperor asked: "How do the five *zang*-organs correspond to nature?"

Uncle Qi answered: "The east is blue. The wood *qi* gets into the liver. The liver opens into the eyes. The essence of wood is stored in the liver. Diseases occur to the head. The sour flavor flows into the liver. The property of the liver is like that of wood.[1] The liver corresponds to the cock and hen in domestic animals, wheat in cereals, *shui* star[2] in the sky, *jiao* (*do*) in musical scales, eight in numbers, and rammish smell in odors.

"So it is known that diseases of the liver affect the sinews.[3]

"The south is red. The fire *qi* gets into the heart. The heart opens into the tongue. The essence of fire is stored in the heart. Diseases occur to the five *zang*-organs. The bitter flavor gets into the heart. The property of the heart is like that of fire. The heart corresponds to the lamb in domestic animals, broomcorn millet in cereals, *ying-huo* star[4] in the sky, *zhi* (*re*) in musical scales, seven in numbers, and burned smell in odors. So it is known that diseases of the heart affect the pulses.[5]

"The center is yellow. The soil *qi* gets into the spleen. The spleen opens into the mouth. The essence of soil is stored in the spleen. Diseases occur at the spine. The sweet flavor gets into the spleen. The property of the spleen is like that of soil. The spleen corresponds to the cattle in domestic animals, millet in cereals, *zhen* star[6] in the sky, *gong* (*mi*) in musical scales, five in numbers, and fragrant smell in odors. So it is known that diseases of the spleen affect the muscles.

"The west is white. The metal *qi* gets into the lungs. The lungs open into the nose. The essence of metal is stored in the lungs. Diseases occur at the back. The acrid flavor gets into the lungs. The property of the lungs is like that of metal. The lungs correspond to the horse in domestic animals, paddy rice in cereals, *tai-bai* star[7] in the sky, *shang* (*so*) in musical scales, nine in numbers, and fishy smell in odors. So it is known that diseases of the lungs affect the skin and body hair.

"The north is black. The water *qi* gets into the kidneys. The kidneys open into the ears. The essence of water is stored in the kidneys. Disease occurs to the small muscles next to the bones. The salty flavor gets into the kidneys. The property of the kidneys is like that of water. The kidneys correspond to the pig in domestic animals, legume in cereals, *chen* star[8] in the sky, *yu* (*la*) in musical scales, six in numbers, and rancid smell in odors. So it is known that diseases of the kidneys affect the bones.

"Thus, an experienced doctor inspects the five *zang*-organs and six *fu*-organs meticulously, considering the favorableness, unfavorableness, *yin*, *yang*, exterior, interior, male and female. All the abstruse information is reviewed mentally. He will not teach unqualified men, nor will he teach incorrect knowledge. These principles are what we should abide by."

Commentary
The foregoing segments depict how the five *zang*-organs correspond to nature, based on the theories of *yin-yang* and the five elements.

The five domestic animals and the five cereals are attributed to the five seasons and the five elements. This suggests that these plants and animals have relationships of inter-promotion or inter-curb during development, which fits ideas in modern biology and ecology.

Annotation
[1] The property of the liver is like that of wood: The liver has a soft consistency. It can be curved or straightened. So, the consistency of the liver is like that of wood.

[2] *Shui* star: It is the essence of wood. It stays at the east, and dominates spring.

[3] It is known that diseases of the liver affect the sinews: The liver dominates the sinews.

[4] *Ying-huo* star: It is the essence of fire. It stays at the south, and dominates summer.

[5] It is known that diseases of the heart affect the pulses: The heart dominates the pulses.

[6] *Zhen* star: It is the essence of soil. It stays at the center, and does not move. It dominates the four seasons.

[7] *Tai-bai* star: It is the essence of metal. It stays at the west, and dominates autumn.

[8] *Chen* star: It is the essence of water. It stays at the north, and dominates winter.

1.3   Sixth Article

Discussion of Separation and Combination of **Yin** *and* **Yang·**
The Plain Questions (*excerpt*)

Original article

The Emperor asked: "I have heard that the sky is *yang*, the earth is *yin*, the sun is *yang*, and the moon is *yin*. 365 days, divided into larger and smaller months, comprise a year. Man is said to correspond to this. But now, there are three couples of *yin* and *yang*. They seem to disobey the rule of a *yin* and a *yang*. Can you explain this?"

Uncle Qi answered: "As to the *yin* and *yang*, the number of them is ten, but ten can be divided into a hundred. To reckon them is a thousand, but a thousand can be separated into ten thousand. Although ten thousand seems an incalculable number, it is entirely based on the rule of a *yin* and a *yang*.

"With the sky above and the earth beneath, what emerges in the soil, but is not exposed to the air is called *yin*-staying, i. e., *yin* within *yin*. What is exposed to the air is called *yang* within *yin*. The *yang* dominates generation, and the *yin* dominates formation. So, generation is due to spring, and growth is due to summer; harvest is due to autumn, and storage is due to winter. Abnormalities may make the heaven and earth blockaded.[1] The changes in the *yin* and *yang* of man are also calculable."

Commentary

This section is a very important part about the *yin* and *yang* in *The Medical Classic of the Yellow Emperor*. It points out the endless divisibility of the *yin* and *yang*. The statement that "the changes in the *yin* and *yang* of man are also calculable" explains that the *yin* and *yang* of man have a certain materialistic basis. The *yang* dominates the generation of living things, and the *yin* governs the formation of living things.

Annotation

[1] Abnormalities may make the heaven and earth blockaded: The heaven and earth may be blockaded in that all changes of generation, growth, harvest, and storage.

Chapter Two
Theory of *Zang*-Organs and Manifestations

The theory of the *zang*-organs and manifestations deals with the physiological functioning of the viscera, their pathogenic changes, and their relationships. It is a very important part of the theoretical system in TCM. The term "*zang*-organs" refers to the viscera, i.e., the five *zang*-organs and six *fu*-organs. The term "manifestations" means the external manifestations of functioning of the viscera.

The theoretical foundation was built upon the experience of many doctors and patients, the practice of medicine, and the knowledge of anatomy, especially the practical application in which the physiological functioning was reflected and proved by the pathologic manifestations and effects of treatment. Accurately speaking, the concept of the *zang*-organs in TCM includes not only the materialistic viscera but also relevant functions. Therefore, simply to equate the *zang*-organs in TCM to the viscera in modern anatomy would be inaccurate.

TCM regards that the complex life's activities of men are the comprehensive functional reflections of the viscera, and that the activities of the *zang*-organs and *fu*-organs are closely cooperative and cannot be separated. So, in addition to the respective functions of the *zang*-*fu* organs, there are close relationships between one *fu*-organ and another *fu*-organ, between one *zang*-organ and another *zang*-organ, between the *zang*-organs and *fu*-organs, and between the *zang*-*fu* organs and external organs and tissues during the course of life's activities. All these have an intimate relationship with natural circumstances.

The major components of this theory include the five *zang*-organs, six *fu*-organs, extremely constant *fu*-organs, essence, spirit, *qi*, blood, fluids, etc. Of these, the five *zang*-organs are the main concerns.

Zang-Organs and *Fu*-Organs

2.1   Ninth Article

Discussion of Zang-Organs and Manifestations
Corresponding to Six · The Plain Questions (excerpt)

Original article

The Emperor asked: "What about the *zang*-organs and their manifestations? "

Uncle Qi answered: "The heart is the basis of life and the room for the spirit. Its bloom is shown on the face. It fills the vessels. It is the greater *yang* within *yang*. The summer *qi* flows into the heart. The lungs are the basis of the *qi* and the room for the *yin* soul.[1] Their bloom is shown on the body hair. They fill the skin. They are the lesser *yin* within *yang*.[2] The autumn *qi* flows into the lungs. The kidneys dominate hibernation. They are the basis of storage and the room for the essence. Their bloom is shown on the hair. They fill the bones. They are the greater *yin* within *yin*.[3] The winter *qi* flows into the kidneys.

"The liver is the basis of resistance to extreme fatigue and the room for the *yang* soul.[4] Its bloom is shown on the nails. It fills the sinews. It is the lesser *yang* within *yin*.[5] The spring *qi* flows into the liver. The spleen, stomach, large intestine, small intestine, triple-warmer and bladder are the basis of garner and the room for the nutritive *qi*.[6] They are called utensils that can transform and transmit foods. Their bloom is shown on the lips. They fill the muscles. They are the type of *yin*-reaching. The soil *qi* flows into them. These above eleven organs are all controlled by the gallbladder.[7]"

Commentary

This section first presents the names of *zang*-organs and *fu*-organs. It then emphasizes the properties of the five *zang*-organs. The article elucidates the functional system of the five *zang*-organs, relating to the five manifested parts of bloom, four seasons, *yin* and *yang*, etc. It reveals the integral idea that man and nature are closely related in TCM. This is one of the basic contents in the theory of the *zang*-organs and manifestations, and also a prominently unique feature in the world medical realm about the relationship between the viscera and nature. The physiological processes and pathogenic changes of the viscera may be shown in the corresponding external body parts.

Through these external manifestations, concrete information about the viscera may be roughly displayed. These manifestations provide reliable evidences for discerning affected places and properties of diseases in diagnosis. For example, as "the kidneys' bloom is shown on the hair, and they fill the bones," if the hair and bones get ill, we could preliminarily diagnose that the kidneys are ill. For another example, the liver is the basis of resistance to extreme fatigue, and its bloom is shown on the nails. In a low fever case that is caused by tiredness, the therapy of nourishing the liver blood has been shown to give a satisfactory result. In clinical practice, the gloss or lack of gloss of the nails can tell the exuberance or debility of the *qi* and blood in the liver channel.

Annotation

[1] The *yin* soul: A soul consists of two parts, i.e., the *yin* part and *yang* part. The *yin* part is called *yin* soul and the *yang* part is called *yang* soul.

[2] They are the lesser *yin* within *yang*: Although the lungs pertain to the greater *yin* in the twelve main channels, they should be the lesser *yin* in the *yang* aspect. The heart and lungs stay above the diaphragm, and all belong to the *yang*. The heart is the greater *yang* within *yang*, while the lungs are the lesser *yin* within *yang*.

[3] They are the greater *yin* within *yin*: Although the kidneys pertain to the lesser *yin* in the twelve main channels, they should be the greater *yin* in the *yin* aspect. The kidneys stay below the diaphragm, and correspond to winter outside.

[4] The *yang* soul: The *yang* part of a soul.

[5] It is the lesser *yang* within *yin*: The liver stays in the abdomen, and corresponds to spring outside.

[6] The nutritive *qi*: When the essential *qi* of water and grains is assimilated at the middle-warmer, the clear part is called nutritive *qi*, which runs inside the vessels; the turbid part is called defensive *qi*, which runs outside the vessels.

[7] These above eleven organs are all controlled by the gallbladder: The gallbladder corresponds to spring. If the spring *qi* rises, all things will be safe. Thus, if the gallbladder *qi* rises, all viscera will be secure. Furthermore, the foot lesser-*yang* gallbladder channel is of half exterior and half interior. The gallbladder is called the upright judiciary official, or an extremely constant *fu*-organ. It can communicate with the *yin* and *yang*. So the other eleven organs are all controlled by it.

2.2   Eighth Article

Discussion of Secret Classic in Ganoderma and Orchid House ·
The Plain Questions (excerpt)

Original article

The Emperor asked: "How do the twelve viscera act? What about their nobleness or humbleness?"

Uncle Qi answered: "A perfect question! Let me remark upon this. The heart is the monarch — thoughts get out there. The lungs are the premier — controls and adjustments get out there.[1] The liver is the general — strategies get out there.[2] The gallbladder is the upright judiciary official — decisions get out there.[3] The pericardium is the herald official — joys and sadness get out there. "The spleen and stomach are the garner officials — the five flavors get out there.

"The large intestine is the transportation official — changes get out there. The small intestine is the reception official — digestions get out there. The kidneys are the power official — skills get out there.[4] The triple-warmer is the water administration official — water networks get out there. The bladder is the water reservation official — fluids are stored there and waste water is discharged after transformation.

"All these twelve organs should keep in balance. Therefore, if the monarch is wise, the subordinates will be safe. Caring for health in this way, a man will enjoy long life without danger, and his world will be prosperous. If the monarch is not wise, the subordinates will be endangered, links of the viscera will be blockaded, and the body will be greatly harmed. Lacking care for health in this bad way, a man's life will be calamitous, and the rule of the monarch will collapse. So, be careful with this!"

Commentary

This section clarifies the main physiological functioning of the viscera and their relationships. The normal running of a country is like that of a body. This comparison is vivid and rational. In this section, the "wise monarch makes the subordinates safe;" and "if the monarch is not wise, the subordinates will be endangered." This explains that the heart plays a leading role in physiological activities of the viscera. All these twelve organs should keep in balance. This viewpoint suggests that the functions of the twelve viscera are separate as well as cooperative. This is one of the important principles of the integral idea of TCM.

Annotation

[1] The lungs are the premier — controls and adjustments get out there: The lungs dominate the *qi*. If the *qi* is harmonious, the viscera will all be congruous. So controls and adjustments get out there.

[2] The liver is the general — strategies get out there: When a man is angry, strategies do not exist.

[3] The gallbladder is the upright judiciary official — decisions get out there: The judiciary official is upright and resolute without hesitation.

[4] The kidneys are the power official — skills get out there: The kidneys dominate the bones. If the bones are strong, the power will be mighty. The kidneys dominate the essence. If a man has not enough essence, he will be unintelligent and have few skills.

2.3 Eleventh Article
Discussion of Differentiations Among the Five Zang*-Organs ·*
The Plain Questions (*excerpt*)

Original article

The Emperor asked: "I have heard that doctors regard the brain and marrow as *zang*-organs, and regard the intestines and stomach as *zang*-organs or as *fu*-organs. When others presented dissent, the doctors insisted on their view. Why did they maintain this opinion?"

Uncle Qi answered: "The brain, marrow, bones, blood vessels, gall-bladder, and womb — these six materials are generated by the earthly *qi*. They all store the *yin*, and their characteristics are like those of the earth. They store things and do not discharge them, and are called extremely constant *fu*-organs. The stomach, large intestine, small intestine, triple-warmer, and bladder — these five materials are generated by the heavenly *qi*. Their characteristics are like those of the heaven. They discharge things and do not store them. They receive the turbid *qi* of the five *zang*-organs, and are called conveyance *fu*-organs. They do not let things stay too long, but convey them away. The anus is controlled by the five *zang*-organs as well. It does not allow things stay there.

"The five *zang*-organs store the essential *qi*, but do not discharge it. So, they are full of essential *qi*, but not full of water and grains. The six *fu*-organs convey things, but do not store them. So, they are full of water and grains, but not full of essential *qi*. When water and grains enter the mouth, they fill the stomach, and the intestines are empty. After that, the intestines are full and the stomach is empty."

Commentary

This section points out that the general function of the five *zang*-organs is storing the essential *qi*, but not discharging it. The five *zang*-organs possess the characteristic of being full of essential *qi*, but not full of water and grains. The general function of the six *fu*-organs is conveying water and grains, but not storing them. The six *fu*-organs have the characteristic of being full of water and grains, but not full of essential *qi*. The extremely constant *fu*-organs are like the six *fu*-organs in their shape, but they are able to store the essential *qi*. The extremely constant *fu*-organs are different from the five *zang*-organs, and also from the six *fu*-organs.

The essential *qi* stored by the five *zang*-organs is the materialistic basis for nutrition of the body, and for all kinds of functional activities. If the essential *qi* is insufficient, not only the five *zang*-organs, but also the six *fu*-organs and their related organs will be affected. So, in clinical practice of treating diseases of the six *fu*-organs and their related organs, one should think about the five *zang*-organs. The six *fu*-organs convey water and grains. The full stomach and empty intestines, and full intestines and empty stomach are the rule of digestion and discharge. In more modern times, the idea that the six *fu*-organs act when being unimpeded was based on the physiological characteristic of discharging, but not of storing things of the six *fu*-organs. In recent years, application of this principle has resulted in easing constipation and loosening the bowels for patients with cases of acute abdominal pain.

What is worth mentioning is that the storage or discharge of the *zang-fu* organs only refers to their respective characteristics of physiological functioning. In fact, there is also turbid *qi* in the five *zang*-organs; and there is essential *qi* in the *fu*-organs. The turbid *qi* in the *zang*-organs is transported by the *fu*-organs. The essential *qi* in the *fu*-organs is stored by the *zang*-organs. In the same way, the characteristic of storing, but of not discharging the essential *qi* of the extremely constant *fu*-organs is not absolute. For example, the gallbladder both stores the bile and dominates its evacuation; the womb both dominates pregnancy and expels menstruation.

In addition, the anus is controlled by the five *zang*-organs, and it does not allow things stay there. This points out the relationship between the anus and the five *zang*-organs in physiology. The opening or closing of the anus is dependent on the domination of the spirit of the heart, the smoothness and arrival of the liver *qi*, the lifting of the spleen *qi*, the diffusion and descent of the lung *qi*, and the astringency of the kidney *qi*. Normal functioning of the anus can adjust ascents and descents of the *qi* of the viscera. So, the normality or abnormality of the functions of the anus can reveal the state of the internal viscera. This possesses certain importance in diagnosis, treatment and prognosis in clinical practice.

2.4   Fifty-fourth Article

Natural Life-Span · The Divine Pivot (*excerpt*)

2.4.1   Original article

The Emperor asked: "In the beginning of one's life, what is the foundation? What is the shield? What is lost that a man will die? What is gained that a man will live?"

Uncle Qi answered: "The mother is the foundation. The father is the shield.[1] One who loses the spirit will die. One who gains the spirit will live."

The Emperor asked: "What is spirit?"

Uncle Qi answered: "The *qi* and blood have been harmonious. The ways of the nutritive *qi* and defensive *qi* have been free. The five *zang*-organs have been formed. The spirit has resided in the heart. The *yang* soul and *yin* soul have been generated. Under these preconditions, a man of sound health will appear."

The Emperor asked: "Men do not all live to be the same age. Some die young and some live long. Some die suddenly. Some experience protracted illness. Why?"

Uncle Qi answered: "The five *zang*-organs are solid. The blood and vessels are harmonious. The muscles are lubricious and flexible. The skin is compact. The running of the nutritive *qi* and defensive *qi* keeps order. Respiration is smooth. The running of the *qi* is in normal proportion to respiration. The six *fu*-organs digest grains. The fluids are well distributed. This man will live long."

The Emperor asked: "How could someone reach a hundred years?"

Uncle Qi answered: "The philtrum is deep and long.[2] The chin is wide and square. The nutritive *qi* and defensive *qi* are congruous. The three parts of the face [3] are prominent. The bones are high and the muscles are plump there. This man will enjoy living to a hundred years without disease."

Annotation

[1] Shield: The "shield" means protection.

[2] The philtrum is deep and long: Chinese people regard this as a symbol of longevity.

[3] The three parts of the face: The face is divided into the upper part, middle part and lower part, which are represented by the forehead, nose and chin.

2.4.2 Original article

The Emperor asked: "What about the waxing and waning of the *qi* from birth to death?"

Uncle Qi answered: "When a man is ten years old, the five *zang*-organs are just stable. The blood and *qi* are unobstructed, and his *qi* mainly stays at the lower part. So, he likes running. When he is twenty years old, the blood and *qi* are blooming, and the muscles are growing. So, he likes trotting. When he is thirty years old, the five *zang*-organs are greatly mature. The muscles are mighty, and the blood vessels are prosperous and full. So, he likes walking. When he is forty, the five *zang*-organs, six *fu*-organs and twelve channels are greatly prosperous and stable. The muscular striae begin to be loosened. The gloss of the skin declines. His hair becomes somewhat hoary. His life reaches its culmination, and he dislikes movements. So, he likes sitting. When he is fifty, the liver *qi* begins to wane. The liver foliage becomes thin. The bile is decreased. The eyes are becoming bleary. When he is sixty, the heart *qi* begins to wane. He suffers from anxiety and sadness, and the blood and *qi* are slumping. So, he likes sleeping. When he is seventy, the spleen *qi* becomes feeble, and the skin dries up. When he is eighty, the lung *qi* becomes weak, and the *yin* soul leaves the body. So, he frequently says things that do not make sense. When he is ninety, the kidney *qi* becomes wizened, and the channels of other four *zang*-organs are nearly empty. When he is a hundred, the five *zang*-organs are completely feeble. The spirit and *qi* are all leaving. Only the body shell exists, and at last he dies."

The Emperor asked: "Why does someone die in middle way?"

Uncle Qi answered: "This is because the man has fragile five *zang*-organs, his philtrum is short, and the nostrils are abnormally open.[1] Gasping and a fulminant disease occur.

"Further, his foundation and fence are weak. The vessels are thin and the blood is scant. His muscles are not solid. The evils of cold and wind attack frequently. His blood and *qi* become feeble. The channels become obstructed. The genuine *qi* and evils conflict with each other. Conversely, the genuine *qi* ushers the evils into the body. So, his life will end in middle way."

Commentary

The above-mentioned two segments explain that the fundamental factors of longevity or short life are both decided by the solidity or fragility of the five *zang*-organs. They emphasize the "inborn base" (kidneys) and further present the theory of inborn endowment, which is based on the idea that "the mother is the foundation and the father is the shield." The theory of inborn endowment provides a theoretical reference to stressing the idea of "caring and cultivating the kidney *qi*" in body building and staving off senility.

Yet, we should notice that the human life span is related not only to inborn factors, but also to care and nourishment after birth, because the spleen and stomach are the "postnatal acquired base." If a man has poor inborn endowment, he may still be nourished to good physique after birth. "The acquired can nourish the inborn." In the meantime, physical exercise may help to prevent exogenous evils from intruding upon the body. The five *zang*-organs are solid. The blood and vessels are harmonious. The essence, *qi* and spirit are vigorous and prosperous.

Thus, one may enjoy long life. The generation of the spirit and its importance to the body exhibit that the essence, *qi* and spirit — these three factors possess relationships of inter-affection. In more recent times, they have been called the "three treasures" of the body. "One who loses the spirit will die, and one who gains the spirit will live." The idea is very significant in clinical observation and pulse-taking. Observing waxing or waning of the spirit of a patient, and feeling the fullness or lack of spirit in the pulses could help to infer the degree of seriousness of a disease, and the favorableness or unfavorableness of prognosis. This is extremely important in diagnosis.

Annotation

[1] The nostrils are abnormally open: The lungs open into the nose. "The nostrils are abnormally open" means that the lung *qi* leaks.

2.5   Fifty-sixth Article

The Five Flavors · The Divine Pivot (*excerpt*)

Original article

The Emperor asked: "How do the five flavor of foods run into the five *zang*-organs?"

Bo Gao answered: "The stomach is the sea of the five *zang*-organs and six *fu*-organs. Water and grains all get into the stomach. The five *zang*-organs and six *fu*-organs are all endowed with *qi* from the stomach. The five flavors run to their favorite *zang*-organs respectively. Sour flavor runs to the liver first. Bitter flavor runs to the heart first. Sweet flavor runs to the spleen first. Acrid flavor runs to the lungs first. Salty flavor runs to the kidneys first. The grain *qi* and fluids keep moving, and the nutritive *qi* and defensive *qi* flow smoothly. Then, egesta are conveyed downward in an orderly fashion."

The Emperor asked: "What about the running of the nutritive *qi* and defensive qi? "

Bo Gao answered: "When grains get into the stomach, the essential *qi* of them first goes to the two warmers where the stomach stays[1] to irrigate the five *zang*-organs. It diverges into two ways, i.e., the way of nutritive *qi*[2] and the way of defensive *qi*.[3] A part of the essential *qi* converging in the chest makes the ancestral *qi*,[4] which constitutes the sea of *qi*. The ancestral *qi* gets out of the lungs through the throat. It is inhaled and exhaled. In regard to the essential *qi* of the heaven and earth,[5] we often see that three kinds are expelled, and only one kind is taken in.[6] So, if a man does not eat for half a day, his *qi* will begin to wane; if he does not eat for a whole day, his *qi* will be poor."

Commentary

This section emphasizes the important roles of the stomach, and presents the view that the stomach is the sea of the five *zang*-organs and six *fu*-organs. Meanwhile, it expounds the relationships among the nutritive *qi*, defensive *qi*, ancestral *qi*, and stomach. The article points out that the essential *qi* of foods is emanated from the middle-warmer to nourish the five *zang*-organs, six *fu*-organs, four limbs and bones. The essential *qi* is separated into two kinds: The clear part is called nutritive *qi*. It runs in the vessels. The turbid part is called defensive *qi*. It runs outside the vessels.

Another part of the essential *qi* that is spread into the chest combines with inhaled air from nature. This combination constitutes the ancestral *qi*. So caring for the stomach *qi* is very important in health care and treatment.

The five flavors of foods have their favorite *zang*-organs respectively. This is the theoretical reference to dietetic treatment. Upon this, the theory of channel tropism of Chinese medicines is developed.

Annotation

[1] The essential *qi* of them first goes to the two warmers where the stomach stays: Above the upper mouth of the stomach is the upper-warmer. The main body of the stomach is at the middle-warmer.

[2] The way of nutritive *qi*: The clear part (relatively soft in property) of the essential *qi* of water and grains is called nutritive *qi*. The nutritive *qi* runs in the way of nutritive *qi*, i.e., the vessels. Thus, the blood is also called nutritive blood.

[3] The way of defensive *qi*: The turbid part (relatively rigid and brave in property) of the essential *qi* of water and grains is called defensive *qi*. The defensive *qi* runs outside the vessels, that is to say, the defensive *qi* runs in the way of defensive *qi*. The defensive *qi* is also called defensive *yang*.

[4] The ancestral *qi*: A part of the essential *qi* that spreads into the chest. It combines with the inhaled clear airs from nature. The combination is ancestral *qi*.

[5] The essential *qi* of the heaven and earth: Here, the essential *qi* of the heaven is air. The essential *qi* of the earth is water and grains.

[6] We often see that three kinds are expelled, and only one kind is taken in: The three kinds are exhaled air, stool and discharged fluids. The one kind is food.

2.6 Thirty-third Article

Discussion of Seas · The Divine Pivot

2.6.1 Original article

The Emperor asked Uncle Qi: "I learned about acupuncture from Confucius.[1] What he talked about was never beyond the nutritive *qi*, defensive *qi*, blood and *qi*. He said that the twelve channels are attributed to the *zang-fu* organs inside, and connect with the limbs outside. Did he bring the twelve channels into correspondences with the four seas?"

Uncle Qi answered: "A man also has four seas. The water of the twelve channels all rushes into the seas. There are four seas in nature. They are the South Sea, West Sea, East Sea and North Sea."

The Emperor asked: "How do these four seas correspond to those of a man?"

Uncle Qi answered: "A man has a sea of marrow, a sea of blood, a sea of *qi*, and a sea of water and grains. These four seas are the counterparts of the natural ones."

The Emperor said: "How far-reaching was the teaching of Confucius where he brought the four seas of men into correspondences with those of nature! What about that?"

Uncle Qi continued: "After we have ascertained the *yin-yang*, exterior-interior, and passing points of the four seas, the four seas could be determined."

The Emperor asked: "Then how do we determine them?"

Uncle Qi answered: "The stomach is the sea of water and grains. Its passing points are from the *qichong* point[2] at the upper part to the *zusanli* point[3] at the lower part.

"The penetrating channel[4] is the sea of the twelve channels. Its passing points are from the *dazhu* point[5] at the upper part to the area of the two *juxu* points[6] at the lower part.

"The chest is the sea of *qi*. Its passing points are from the *yamen* point[7] and *dazhui* point[8] at the upper part to the *renying* point[9] at the front side.

"The brain is the sea of marrow. Its passing points are from the *bai-hui* point[10] at the vertex down to the *fengfu* point.[11]"

Annotation

[1] Confucius: A great ideologist of the ancient times, for whom Confucianism is named.

[2] The *qichong* point: Also known as ST – 30 who, i.e., *Qi* Thoroughfare. It pertains to the foot bright-*yang* stomach channel, five thumb-widths below the navel, two thumb-widths away from the ventral medial line. (The thumb-width is a variable unit of measurement equivalent to the patient's thumb-width. Doctors often use the patient's thumb-width to determine acupuncture points.)

[3] The *zusanli* point: Also known as ST – 36 who, i.e., Foot Three *Li*. It pertains to the foot bright-*yang* stomach channel, a bit more than three thumb-widths below the lower edge of the kneecap, at the front edge of the lateral face of the shank. It is a transverse-finger away from the front edge of the shin.

[4] The penetrating channel: One of the eight peculiar channels. It starts from the lower abdomen, gets out of the perineum, and goes up inside the spine. Its main lines run up along both sides of the abdomen, reach the throat, and run around the lips.

[5] The *dazhu* point: Also known as BL – 11 who, i.e., Great Shuttle. It pertains to the foot greater-*yang* bladder channel under the spinal process of the first thoracic vertebra, about one and a half thumb-widths away from the back media line.

[6] The two *juxu* points: Include the *shangjuxu* point (ST – 37 who, i.e., Upper Great Hollow) and *xiajuxu* point (ST – 39 who, i.e., Lower Great Hollow). The *shangjuxu* point is three thumb-widths below the *zusanli* point. The *xiajuxu* point is three thumb-widths below the *shangjuxu* point. They pertain to the foot bright-*yang* stomach channel.

[7] The *yamen* point: Also known as GV – 15 who, i.e., Mute's Gate. It pertains to the governing channel that is one of the eight peculiar channels, a half thumb-width just above the back edge of the hair, on the back medial line of the head.

[8] The *dazhui* point: Also known as GV – 14 who, i.e., Great Hammer. It pertains to the governing channel, just below the seventh cervical vertebra.

[9] The *renying* point: ST – 9 who, i.e., Man's Prognosis. It is one and a half thumb-widths away and beside the Adam's apple, pertaining to the foot bright-*yang* stomach channel.

[10] The *baihui* point: Also known as GV – 20 who, i.e., Hundred Convergences. It pertains to the governing channel, on the top of the head.

[11] The *fengfu* point: Also known as GV – 16 who, i.e., Wind House. It pertains to the governing channel, one thumb-width just above the back edge of the hair, on the back medial line of the head.

2.6.2 Original article

The Emperor asked: "What things are advantageous and pernicious to the four seas? How do they cause a man to survive or to fail to survive?"

Uncle Qi answered: "Favorableness causes one to survive and unfavorableness causes one to fail to survive. Knowing how to make adjustment is advantageous and not knowing is pernicious."

The Emperor asked: "What about the favorableness and unfavorableness of the four seas?"

Uncle Qi answered: "If the sea of *qi* is surplus,[1] the *qi* will be full in the chest, and a man will feel his chest stuffy and have a red face. If the sea of *qi* is deficient,[2] he will be too listless to speak due to the scant *qi*. If the sea of blood is surplus, a man will always feel his body big and not be able to feel his hidden chronic diseases. If the sea of blood is deficient, he will always feel his body small and not be able to feel his hidden chronic diseases too. If the sea of water and grains is surplus, a man will feel his abdomen full. If the sea of water and grains is deficient, he will have no desire for food, even in hunger. If the sea of marrow is surplus, a man will be more sinewy and agile than others.[3] If the sea of marrow is deficient, he will have dizziness, tinnitus, weary limbs, blindness, listlessness, and drowsiness."

The Emperor asked: "I have known the favorableness and unfavorableness of the four seas. Then, how can we adjust them?"

Uncle Qi answered: "By detecting their connecting points, and adjusting their deficiencies or surpluses without violating rules. Obedience is helpful to recovery, and disobedience is doomed to fail."

The Emperor praised: "Marvelous!"

Commentary

This section explains that the stomach, penetrating channel, chest, and brain are the converging places of water and grains, blood, *qi*, and marrow. The four seas of the body resemble the four seas in nature. It points out that the four seas are very important in life's activities. The connecting points and symptoms due to surplus and deficiency are also discussed.

The symptoms due to surplus and deficiency are essentially related to disorders of the *zang-fu* organs, such as the lungs, stomach, kidneys, etc. This is often seen in clinical practice.

Take the deficiencies as examples. "If the sea of *qi* is deficient, a man will be too listless to speak due to the scant *qi*." This condition is closely related to the shortage of the kidney *qi*. "If the sea of water and grains is deficient, a man will have no desire for food, even in hunger." This condition is closely related to the weakness of *qi* of the stomach and spleen. "If the sea of marrow is deficient, a man will have dizziness, tinnitus, weary limbs, blindness, listlessness, and drowsiness." This condition is closely pertinent to the deficiency of the kidney *yin*.

Annotation
[1] Surplus: Evils are surplus.

[2] Deficient: The genuine right *qi* is deficient.

[3] If the sea of marrow is surplus, a man will be more sinewy and agile than others: In all mentioned eight conditions, only this one is not pathogenic.

2.7 Second Article

Basic Points · The Divine Pivot (*excerpt*)

Original article

The lungs act reciprocally with the large intestine. The large intestine is the conveyance *fu*-organ. The heart acts reciprocally with the small intestine. The small intestine is the reception *fu*-organ. The liver acts reciprocally with the gallbladder. The gallbladder is the bilious *fu*-organ. The spleen acts reciprocally with the stomach. The stomach is the five-cereals *fu*-organ. The kidneys act reciprocally with the bladder. The bladder is the fluid *fu*-organ. The lesser-*yin* kidney channel pertains to the kidneys. The kidneys connect with the lungs through the lesser-*yin* kidney channel. So the kidneys command the bladder and lungs. The triple-warmer is the water administration *fu*-organ. Water networks get out there. The triple-warmer is the solitary *fu*-organ without a counterpart. These are the correspondences of the six *fu*-organs and five *zang*-organs.

Commentary

This section describes the physiological functioning of the six *fu*-organs, and the intrinsic interior-exterior linkages of the six *fu*-organs and five *zang*-organs. Due to the physiological correspondences of the *zang*-organs and *fu*-organs, the counterparts can affect each other's pathology. So, in clinical practice we could treat the *zang*-organs when the *fu*-organs are ill, and we could treat the *fu*-organs when the *zang*-organs are ill, for instance, when the lung *qi* fails to emanate, when there are cough and gasping, and when the patient is constipated. In the treatment, easing constipation could help to emanate the lung *qi*; on the other hand, emanating the lung *qi* and moistening the lungs could help to ease constipation. In another case, when bedwetting occurs due to failed bladder restraint, warming the kidney *yang* usually results in a satisfactory effect.

"The lesser-*yin* kidney channel pertains to the kidneys. The kidneys connect with the lungs through the lesser-*yin* kidney channel. So, the kidneys command the bladder and lungs." This explains that the lungs and kidneys are connected by the lesser-*yin* kidney channel in structure. On the other hand, speaking about the function, the kidneys dominate water and the lungs are the upper source of water. So, these two organs play very important roles in the internal water metabolism. Under pathogenic conditions, diseases of the lungs could affect the kidneys, and diseases of the kidneys could influence the lungs.

The view has been presented that the lungs should be treated in nephritis, based on the foregoing theory. In addition, in a case of gasping, the therapy of nourishing the kidneys to draw in the *qi* is sometimes efficacious.

2.8   Twenty-ninth Article

Discussion of Greater- Yin *and Bright-* Yang·
The Plain Questions

2.8.1   Original article

The Emperor asked: "The greater-*yin* spleen channel acts reciprocally with the bright-*yang* stomach channel. Why do they have different symptoms of illness?"

Uncle Qi answered: "The two channels have different locations. They alternate vacuity and repletion, and favorableness and unfavorableness in the four seasons.[1] They are respectively attributed to a *zang*-organ and a *fu*-organ. Different attributes determine different diseases."

The Emperor said: "I want to hear about these differences."

Uncle Qi explained: "The *yang qi* of the body is bestowed by the heavenly *qi*. It dominates the exterior. The *yin qi* of the body is bestowed by the earthly *qi*. It dominates the interior. The exogenous attacks are usually due to surplus evils, and the internal injuries are usually due to the deficient right *qi*. So, when bandit wind[2] and evils come, the *yang* is attacked first; intemperate diet and irregular life cause the *yin* to be stricken first. The exogenous evils get into the six *fu*-organs through the *yang* channels. The injuries caused by intemperate diet and chaotic life affect the five *zang*-organs through the *yin* channels. The affected six *fu*-organs show pyretic body, abnormal sleep patterns and gasping. The affected five *zang*-organs reveal abdominal fullness and blockade, diarrhea containing undigested foods, even to the point where the stool contains pus and blood. So, the larynx dominates the heavenly *qi*,[3] and the pharynx dominates the earthly *qi*.[4]

"Hence, the *yang* parts are easy to be attacked by wind evil, and the *yin* parts are easy to be stricken by damp evil. So, the *yin qi* runs from the feet to the head, then moves down to the fingers along the arms. The *yang qi* runs from the fingers to the head, then moves down to the feet. So we say: Disorders due to *yang* evils are at the upper part, and they will move down with the *qi* after a long time; disorders due to *yin* evils are at the lower part, and they will move up with the *qi* after a long time. Therefore, wind evil assails the top first, and damp evil assails the bottom first."

Annotation

[1] They alternate vacuity and repletion, and favorableness and unfavorableness in the four seasons: In spring and summer, the bright-*yang* is replete, and the greater-*yin* is vacuous. In autumn and winter, the bright-*yang* is vacuous, and the greater-*yin* is replete. In spring and summer, the bright-*yang* is favorable, and the greater-*yin* is unfavorable. In autumn and winter, the bright-*yang* is unfavorable, and the greater-*yin* is favorable.

[2] Bandit wind: Literally, wind evil like a bandit.

[3] The larynx dominates the heavenly *qi*: The larynx dominates respiration because it is where the lung *qi* gets out.

[4] The pharynx dominates the earthly *qi*: Water and grains enter the stomach through the pharynx.

2.8.2 Original article

The Emperor asked: "Why do the four limbs fail to move freely when the spleen gets ill? "

Uncle Qi answered: "The four limbs are endowed with *qi* from the stomach. If the *qi* fails to reach the channels, it is due to disorders of the spleen, which dominates the endowment. Now, when the spleen is ill, it cannot move fluids for the stomach. The four limbs cannot receive *qi* from water and grains. The *qi* weakens day after day. The blood vessels become impeded. The tendons, bones and muscles cannot be nourished by the *qi*. So, the four limbs fail to move at will."

The Emperor asked: "Why is that the spleen does not dominate an independent season?"

Uncle Qi answered: "The spleen pertains to soil. It dominates the center. The other four *zang*-organs dominate the four seasons respectively. The spleen dominates the middle eighteen days in every season. It does not dominate an independent season. The spleen always manifests the essence of stomach soil noticeably. The soil generates everything and takes the rules of the heaven and earth. The spleen *qi* reaches the head and feet, up and down. The spleen does not dominate an independent season."

The Emperor asked: "The spleen connects with the stomach by membranes. How can the spleen move fluids[1] for the stomach? "

Uncle Qi answered: "The foot greater-*yin* spleen channel is the third *yin* channel.[2] Its line connects with the stomach, spleen and throat. So, the spleen moves *qi* in the three *yin* channels for the stomach. The stomach dominates the exterior. It is the sea of the five *zang*-organs and six *fu*-organs. The spleen also moves *qi* in the three *yang* channels for the stomach. All the organs are endowed with *qi* from the stomach through their channels."

Commentary

The discussion of this article focuses on the relationship between the greater-*yin* spleen channel and bright-*yang* stomach channel. Concerning their structure, the spleen and stomach are connected by membranes, and they are linked by their channels. Concerning their physiology, the stomach dominates decomposition of food, and the spleen dominates digestion. The decomposition by the stomach is the preparation for the digestion by the spleen, and the digestion is also the continuance of the decomposition. The close relationship between the stomach and spleen plays a very important directive role in clinical practice. Harmonious stomach *qi* guarantees the source of nutrients. The healthy spleen guarantees the transmission of essence of water and grains. So, fortifying the spleen and stomach is an important way to heal internal injuries.

The spleen dominates the four extremities. If the spleen becomes ill and cannot move fluids for the stomach, the four limbs will fail to move at will. So in clinical practice, a case characterized by feeble limbs and lack of free movement, or muscular atrophy of the limbs, may be caused by the spleen and stomach. *The Discussion of Atrophy Diseases*, an article in *The Plain Questions*, presents the therapeutic rule of "exclusively selecting the bright-*yang* stomach in atrophy diseases." It was most likely based on the idea.

What is notable is that "the soil generates everything and takes the rules of the heaven and earth." It emphasizes the idea of "taking the spleen and stomach seriously." The famous ancient doctor, Li Dongyuan, who wrote the eminent work *Discussion on the Spleen and Stomach*, was greatly enlightened by this thought. He was one of the four great medical masters in the Jin-Yuan Period (1115 — 1368). This sect of doctors represented by him is respectfully called Soil-Enriching School.

"The spleen does not dominate an independent season. It dominates the middle eighteen days in every season." This is another view about the correspondences of the five *zang*-organs and the four seasons. In the former view, the spleen dominates late summer.

"Wind evil assails the top first, and damp evil assails the bottom first." This explains the pathogenic characteristics of wind evil and damp evil.

Annotation

[1] Fluids: In this context, mean the essential *qi* of water and grains.

[2] The foot greater-*yin* spleen channel is the third *yin* channel: The cold-*yin* is the first *yin* channel. The lesser-*yin* is the second *yin* channel. The greater-*yin* is the third *yin* channel.

2.9   Twenty-first Article

Discussion of Differentiations Among the Channels ·
The Plain Questions (*excerpt*)

Original article

After grains enter the stomach, the essential *qi* is spread into the liver, and its other part nourishes the sinews. After foods get into the stomach, the dense part of the *qi* gets into the heart, and its other part nourishes the blood vessels. The *qi* runs in the channels and flows into the lungs. The lungs face the hundred vessels, and push the essential *qi* into the skin and body hair. The *qi* and blood combine and run in the channels normally. Then, the *qi* and blood get into the other four *zang*-organs. The *qi* keeps in balance, and manifests its state at the wrist pulse with concentration. Death and life could be detected here.

After water gets into the stomach, the essential *qi* of water spills and is transported upward to the spleen. The spleen continues to push it upward to the lungs.[1] The lungs dredge the water ways and transmit the water *qi* downward to the bladder.[2] The essential *qi* of water spreads everywhere and runs into the channels of the five *zang*-organs. Conforming to the rules of the four seasons, five *zang*-organs and *yin-yang*, all functions cooperate.

Commentary

This section describes the two ways that the essential *qi* of water and grains is transported. It also illuminates the theory and value of taking the wrist pulse in diagnosis. It sets up the theoretical foundation that pulse-taking can diagnose diseases of the viscera.

In this section, "the essential *qi* of water spills and is transported upward to the spleen, and the spleen continues to push it upward to the lungs." It is the theoretical basis for the methods of "cultivating the soil to promote the metal" and "reducing phlegm to treat the spleen." "The lungs dredge the water ways and transmit water *qi* downward to the bladder." This is the theoretical source of the ideas that "the lungs are the upper source of water" and that one should "treat the lungs in edema."

Annotation

[1] After water gets into the stomach, the essential *qi* of water spills and is transported upward

to the spleen. The spleen continues to push it upward to the lungs: When water enters the stomach, the essential *qi* is transported to the spleen first. This description suggests that the middle-warmer acts like a fermenting spot. The spleen pushes the essential *qi* upward to the lungs. This description suggests that the earthly *qi* is steamed and ascends to be clouds and the upper-warmer acts like a mist.

[2] The lungs dredge the water ways and transmit the water *qi* downward to the bladder: The lungs correspond to the heaven and govern the *qi*. So, they can dredge the water ways and transmit the water *qi* downward to the bladder. The earthly *qi* ascends to be clouds and the heavenly *qi* descends to be rain.

2.10   Seventeenth Article

Measurements of the Channels · The Divine Pivot (excerpt)

Original article

The five *zang*-organs connect with the upper orifices through their channels. So, the lung *qi* opens into the nose. If the lungs are harmonious, the nose can smell both fragrant and foul odors. The heart *qi* opens into the tongue. If the heart is harmonious, the tongue can taste the five flavors. The liver *qi* opens into the eyes. If the liver is harmonious, the eyes can distinguish the five colors. The spleen *qi* opens into the mouth. If the spleen is harmonious, the mouth can distinguish the five cereals. The kidney *qi* opens into the ears. If the kidneys are harmonious, the ears can hear the five musical scales. If the five *zang*-organs are out of harmony, the functioning of the seven orifices will be impeded. If the six *fu*-organs are out of harmony, carbuncles will appear.[1]

Commentary

This section explains that the upper seven orifices are endowed with the essential *qi* from the five *zang*-organs to support their normal physiological functioning. It is the theoretical source of the idea that "the five *zang*-organs dominate the five sense organs." When the five *zang*-organs are ill, symptoms are shown in the corresponding sense organs. For example, the heat of the liver causes bloodshot eyes; the deficiency of the kidneys creates tinnitus; the heat of the spleen creates a sweet taste in the mouth; a blazing fire of the heart causes an inflamed tongue; impeded lung *qi* causes a stuffy nose, and so on. Therefore, when the five sense organs are ill, treatment can be begun with the five *zang*-organs.

Annotation

[1] If the six *fu*-organs are out of harmony, carbuncles will appear: The six *fu*-organs pertain to the *yang* and dominate the exterior. Carbuncles are *yang* signs. If the six *fu*-organs are out of harmony, the *qi* and blood will be stagnant. Stagnation can induce heat. Heat may make the muscles rotten. Then carbuncles appear.

2.11   Eightieth Article

Discussion of Great Puzzlement · The Divine Pivot (*excerpt*)

Original article

The essential *qi* of the five *zang*-organs and six *fu*-organs all flows into the eyes to obtain visual sense. The eyes are the nests of the visceral essences.

The essence of the kidneys nourishes the pupils. The essence of the liver nourishes the colored parts of the eyes (irises). The essence of the heart nourishes the capillaries. The essence of the lungs nourishes the whites of the eyes (conjunctivae). The essence of the spleen nourishes the eyelids. The pupils, colored parts, whites, capillaries and concerned channels constitute a visual system that connects with the brain upward and gets out of the center of the back of the neck.

Commentary

This section discusses the physiological links between the eyes and the five *zang*-organs. The pupils pertain to the kidneys. The colored parts pertain to the liver. The capillaries pertain to the heart. The whites pertain to the lungs. The eyelids pertain to the spleen. This idea was the theoretical foundation of "the theory of five wheels" in ophthalmology in later times. The theory of five wheels regards the pupil as a water wheel, the white as a *qi* wheel, the iris as a wind wheel, the capillaries as a blood wheel, and the eyelids as a muscle wheel. The five wheels respectively connect with the kidneys, lungs, liver, heart and spleen. This theory is very important in helping to diagnose and treat diseases of the eyes. For example, the method of "invigorating the spleen and enriching the *qi*" could be used to treat prolapse of the eyelids due to spleen deficiency. When the capillaries penetrate the irises, it is likely due to a blazing fire of the lungs affecting the liver. The method of "cooling the lungs and nourishing the liver" is usually effective.

Essence, *Qi* and Spirit

2.12   Thirtieth Article

Decisive Qi · The Divine Pivot

2.12.1   Original article

The Emperor asked: "I was told that men have essence, *qi*, liquid, fluids, blood and vessels. I think they are all the same substance, but have six different names, though I don't know why."

Uncle Qi answered: "Two sexes wrestle and mix, a body form is then made. What has been generated before the body is generated is called essence (i.e., sperm or ovum)."

"What is *qi*?"

Uncle Qi answered: "The upper-warmer emanates and spreads the essential *qi* of the five cereals. What nourishes the skin, fills the body and moistens the body hair like irrigation of mist and dew, is called *qi*."

"What is liquid?[1]"

Uncle Qi replied: "Sweat discharged from the muscular striae is called liquid."

"What are fluids?"

Uncle Qi answered: "After grains get in, the *qi* becomes full. What spills into the bones to aid flexibility and stretching, what exudes to nourish the brain and marrow, and what moistens and lubricates the skin, are called fluids."

"What is blood?"

Uncle Qi answered: "After the middle-warmer is endowed with *qi*, filtered and purified water becomes red. It is called blood."

"What are vessels?"

Uncle Qi answered: "What restrain the nutritive blood to make it run in them are called vessels."

Annotation

[1] Liquid: In this context, refers to sweat. There are five kinds of metabolic liquids in all, including sweat, urine, saliva, tears and water (that causes edema).

2.12.2   Original article

The Emperor asked: "How could we know the surpluses or shortages of these six kinds of substances, the amount of the *qi*, deficient or replete brain and marrow, and the clearness or turbidity of the blood and vessels?"

Uncle Qi answered: "Loss of the essence makes deafness. Loss of the *qi* makes bleary eyes. Loss of the liquid makes the muscular striae open and makes the sweat profuse. Loss of the fluids makes it inconvenient to flex and stretch the joints. The loss makes the sheen of the skin wizened, the brains reduced, the shanks feeble, and frequently causes tinnitus. Loss of the blood makes the skin pale and colorless. Loss of the vessel *qi* makes the pulse empty and weak."

The Emperor asked: "What about nobleness and humbleness of these six kinds of substances?"

Uncle Qi answered: "These six kinds are dominated by regular masters respectively.[1] The nobleness or humbleness and normality or abnormality are controlled by their masters. However, they are all produced from the five cereals, and the stomach is still the great sea."

Commentary

This article chiefly talks about the generation and functioning of the essence (i.e., sperm or ovum), *qi*, liquid, fluids, blood and vessels. The main symptoms produced by great losses of these substances are also covered. These provide a reference to "ascertaining causes from symptoms and treating according to causes" in clinical practice. For example, a pale and colorless face expresses a loss of blood, so blood tonics should be used.

On the other hand, these six kinds of substances have close relationships and can affect each other. To illustrate, a great loss of blood usually concurs with an injury to the fluids; a great loss of sweat usually concurs with a blood deficiency. So we must notice the mutual affect of the "liquid and fluide" and the "*qi* and blood" in clinical practice. The primary factor and secondary factor should be determined. The correct treatment then can be adopted.

Furthermore, "these six kinds are dominated by regular masters respectively" and "the stomach is still the great sea." These ideas somewhat possess the thought of dialectics. Though these six substances can be combined into a single entity, they pertain to different masters. The essence pertains to the kidneys. The *qi* belongs to the lungs. The liquid and fluids pertain to the spleen. The blood pertains to the liver. The vessels pertain to the heart.

We must not only look at the mutual affects among the six substances but also notice the respectively tendentious relationships between these six substances and the five *zang*-organs. We cannot ignore that the stomach is the source of these six substances. So replenishing the spleen and stomach is of almost inestimable value in treating deficiencies of these six substances in clinical practice.

Annotation

[1] These six kinds are dominated by regular masters respectively: The kidneys dominate the essence. The lungs dominate the *qi*. The spleen dominates the liquid and fluids. The liver dominates the blood. The heart dominates the vessels.

2.13   Eighteenth Article

Generation and Meeting of Nutritive Qi and
Defensive Qi · The Divine Pivot

Original article

The Emperor asked: "How is a man endowed with *qi*? How do the *yin* and *yang* meet? What is nutritive *qi*? What is defensive *qi*? Where does the nutritive *qi* come from? Where does the defensive *qi* meet the nutritive *qi*? The *qi* of old men is different from that of young men. The *qi* runs in different routes by day and by night. How do the nutritive *qi* and defensive *qi* meet? "

Uncle Qi answered: "Men are endowed with *qi* from grains. When grains get into the stomach, the *qi* is transported to the lungs. Then, the five *zang*-organs and six *fu*-organs are all endowed with *qi*. The clear part of the *qi* is called nutritive *qi*. The turbid part of the *qi* is called defensive *qi*. The nutritive *qi* runs inside the vessels. The defensive *qi* runs outside the vessels. Both move endlessly and meet once after fifty circles. In the way of a *yin* channel and a *yang* channel, the circulation of the nutritive *qi* and defensive *qi* is ceaseless, in a loop. The defensive *qi* runs twenty-five circles in the night, and the other twenty-five circles in the day. So, when the defensive *qi* reaches the *yang*, the person wakes up. When the defensive *qi* arrives at the *yin*, the person goes to sleep. So we say: The *yang* reaches its climax at the midday. It is called double-*yang*. The *yin* reaches its climax at midnight. It is called double-*yin*.

"So the greater-*yin* lung channel dominates the interior (i.e., nutritive *qi*), and the greater-*yang* bladder channel dominates the exterior[1] (i.e., defensive *qi*). The nutritive *qi* and defensive *qi* respectively run twenty-five circles in the day and the other twenty-five circles in the night. The midnight is double-*yin*. The *yin* begins to decline after midnight, and vanishes at dawn. Then, the *yang* begins to increase. The midday is double-*yang*. The *yang* begins to decline after that, and vanishes at dusk. Then, the *yin* begins to increase. At midnight, the nutritive *qi* and defensive *qi* meet in the viscera, while people are all sleeping. This is called midnight meeting. The *yin* vanishes at dawn, and then the *yang* begins to increase. The nutritive *qi* and defensive *qi* circulate through the day and night, like the endless running of the sun and moon."

The Emperor asked: "Why don't old men want to sleep in the night? Why don't young men want to sleep in the day?"

Uncle Qi answered: "Young men have exuberant *qi* and blood. The muscles are lubricious. The ways of their *qi* are smooth. The nutritive *qi* and defensive *qi* run normally. So, young men are spirited in the daytime and sleep well at night. Old men have debilitated *qi* and blood. The muscles are desiccated. The ways of their *qi* are uneven. The functions of the five *zang*-organs are not congruous. The nutritive *qi* is weak. The defensive *qi* is poor and competes with the nutritive *qi* for complement. So, old men are not spirited in the daytime and do not sleep well at night."

The Emperor asked: "Where do the nutritive *qi* and defensive *qi* come from?"

Uncle Qi answered: "The nutritive *qi* comes from the middle-warmer. The defensive *qi* comes from the lower-warmer."

The Emperor asked: "Can you please tell me the functions of the *qi* of the upper-warmer (i.e., ancestral *qi*)?"

Uncle Qi answered: "The *qi* of the upper-warmer comes from the upper mouth of the stomach. It ascends along the esophagus, penetrates across the diaphragm, and spreads in the chest. It reaches the armpit, runs along the hand greater-*yin* lung channel, and returns to the hand bright-*yang* large-intestine channel. Then, it goes up to the tongue, and runs down to the foot bright-*yang* stomach channel. The ancestral *qi* runs together with the nutritive *qi* twenty-five circles in the day and the other twenty-five circles in the night.[2] After fifty circles, the ancestral *qi* prosperously meets at the hand greater-*yin* lung channel."

The Emperor asked: "Somebody has just eaten hot food. Before the essential *qi* of food is generated, the man sweats on the face, back, or half part of the body. The sweat does not run in the normal ways of the defensive *qi*, and gets out. What is the reason?"

Uncle Qi answered: "This is because the man is assailed by exogenous wind evil. His skin and body hair are steamed by wind and heat. Then, the muscular striae are forced open and the sweat escapes. So, the sweat does not run in the normal ways of the defensive *qi*. The sweat *qi* is brave, slippery and swift. When the muscular striae open, the sweat gets out and does not run through the normal ways of the defensive *qi*. Thus, the disease is called sweat-leakage."

The Emperor asked: "Can you please tell me the functions of the *qi* of the middle-warmer?"

Uncle Qi answered: "The *qi* of the middle-warmer stays at the middle part of the abdomen under the upper-warmer. The middle-warmer receives the essential *qi* of foods. It discards dross, purifies fluids, and transports them to the vessels of the lungs. There, they become blood to nourish the body. Nothing is more valuable than the blood. Thus, it is exclusively permitted to run in the channels. It is called nutritive *qi*."

The Emperor asked: "What does it mean that the blood and *qi* with different names are of the same kind?"

Uncle Qi answered: "The nutritive *qi* and defensive *qi* are the essential *qi* of food. The blood that is turned red by the heart spirit is the purified fluid of the middle-warmer. So, the nutritive *qi*, defensive *qi* and blood, although having different names, are homologous. Therefore, one whose blood is despoiled has no sweat, and one whose sweat is despoiled has no blood. So, if a man has despoliation of both blood and sweat, he will die; if a man has despoliation of only blood or sweat, he will survive."

The Emperor asked: "Can you please tell me the functions of the *qi* of the lower-warmer?"

Uncle Qi answered: "The *qi* of the lower-warmer flows into the ileum and rushes into the bladder. So, water and grains usually stay in the stomach, and then the dregs get down the large intestine. The small intestine filters and purifies water and grains, and then the wastewater seeps into the bladder along the lower-warmer.[3]"

The Emperor asked: "A man drinks some wine. The wine also gets into the stomachwith the food. Why is the urine expelled before the food is digested?"

Uncle Qi answered: "Wine is liquid of cooked cereals. Its property is strong and slippery. So, even getting into the stomach later than the cereals, the wine gets out earlier."

The Emperor said: "Good! That is why I heard that the upper-warmer is like a mist, the middle-warmer is like a ferment spot, and the lower-warmer is like a sluice.[4] That is the answer!"

Commentary

This article mainly discusses the generation, functioning, running and meeting of the nutritive *qi* and defensive *qi*. Although the nutritive *qi* and defensive *qi* are all generated from the essential *qi* of foods, they have different functions. The nutritive *qi* runs in the vessels. It has the nutritive function, and dominates internal guarding. The defensive *qi* runs outside the vessels. It has the defensive function around the body like a fence. The nutritive *qi* begins to run from the hand greater-*yin* lung channel, moves along the twelve channels, and returns to the hand greater-*yin* lung channel at dawn. The defensive *qi* starts to run from the foot greater-*yang* bladder channel, moves inside the *yang* channels in the daytime, and runs inside the five *zang*-organs at night. It returns to the greater-*yang* bladder channel at dawn. The nutritive *qi* and defensive *qi* meet in the viscera between 23:00 and 01:00. The circulations are endless.

In this article, we learn that "one whose blood is despoiled has no sweat, and one whose sweat is despoiled has no blood." This idea is a relatively large enlightenment to treatment. For example, the medical book, *Discussion on Damage from Cold*, presented the admonishment that "one who has nosebleeds cannot be promoted perspiration" and "one who has skin ulcers cannot be promoted perspiration." In clinical practice, if one with deficiency or loss of blood is attacked by exogenous evils, diaphoresis should be promoted by nourishing the *yin* and enriching the blood. The theory that "the blood and sweat are homologous" developed from this idea.

Annotation

[1] The greater-*yin* lung channel dominates the interior (i.e., nutritive *qi*), and the greater-*yang* bladder channel dominates the exterior (i.e., defensive *qi*): This is because the nutritive *qi* begins to run from the greater-*yin* lung channel, and at its finish returns there. The defensive *qi* begins to run from the greater-*yang* bladder channel, and at its finish returns there.

[2] The ancestral *qi* runs together with the nutritive *qi* twenty-five circles in the day and the other twenty-five circles in the night: The nutritive *qi* is pushed forward by the ancestral *qi* to run in the body. Though the nutritive *qi* is generated at the middle-warmer, it is pushed ahead by the *qi* of the upper-warmer.

[3] The small intestine filters and purifies water and grains, and then the wastewater seeps into the bladder along the lower-warmer: The small intestine receives water and grains, which are decomposed by the stomach. After filtration and purification, the clear part and turbid part are detached. The clear part, i.e., essential *qi*, is assimilated to nourish the body. The turbid part, i.e., dregs and wastewater, are transported into the large intestine and bladder.

[4] That is why I heard that the upper-warmer is like a mist, the middle-warmer is like a fer-

ment spot, and the lower-warmer is like a sluice: These are used to describe the functions of the triple-warmer. The heart and lungs that stay at the upper-warmer spread the essential *qi* as if a mist permeates and irrigates the body. The spleen and stomach staying at the middle-warmer decompose and digest foods and assimilate the essential *qi* as if a ferment spot is working. The kidneys and bladder staying at the lower-warmer discharge water like a sluice.

2.14   Thirty-sixth Article

Differentiations Among Five Metabolic Liquids · The Divine Pivot

Original article

The Emperor asked: "Water and grains enter the mouth. They are transported to the intestines and stomach. Then, their water is excreted in five ways. When the weather is cold and a man is thinly clad, the discharged water is urine and steam. When the weather is hot and the clothes are thick, it is sweat. When a man is excessively sorrowful, the discharged water is tears. When the spleen and stomach are hot, their functions become abnormal and much saliva is excreted. When evils intrude, the *qi* gets obstructed and stagnant, and water distention ensues. What are the reasons?"

Uncle Qi answered: "Water and grains all enter the mouth. The five flavors of them rush into their own seas respectively.[1] The fluids run in their respective ways. So the triple-warmer transports the *qi* .[2] What warm the muscles and fill the skin are active fluids. What stay and do not move are inactive fluids. When the weather is hot and the clothes are thick, the muscular striae open and sweat comes out. If cold stays in the muscles, the accumulated foam will induce pain.[3] When the weather is cold, the muscular striae remain closed. The *qi* is uneven and stands still, then water gets down into the bladder. So the discharged water is urine and steam.

"Respecting the five *zang*-organs, six *fu*-organs and other organs, the heart is the monarch; the ears dominate hearing; the eyes dominate vision; the lungs are the premier; the liver is the general; the spleen is the guard;[4] the kidneys govern the exterior.[5]

"So, the fluids of the five *zang*-organs and six *fu*-organs all seep upward into the eyes. If one is greatly sorrowful, the heart system[6] gets spasmodic. Spasms make the lungs feel lifted. The 'lifted' lungs make the fluids exude upward. The heart system and lungs cannot stay at the normal places. The *qi* abruptly goes up and suddenly goes down, coughing occurs, and tears flow. If the stomach and spleen are hot, rapid digestion happens and worms[7] run up and down. The intestines and stomach become dilated with gas, and the functioning of the stomach becomes abnormal. The stomach *qi* adversely flows upward; thus much saliva is excreted.

"A part of the fluids from the five cereals is mixed into ointment, which exudes into the bones nourishing the brain and marrow, and flowing downward to the groin.

"If the *yin* and *yang* are uncoordinated,[8] this kind of fluids spills and flows downward to the genital area. The fluids of the marrow decrease and flow downward. Too much of this can induce deficiency.

"The deficiency may cause painful back and loins and feeble shanks. The ways of the fluids become impeded. The four seas become obstructed. The triple-warmer is not able to transport water. The fluids fail to be transformed. Water and grains move into the stomach and intestines together, and are amassed in the ileum. Water stays at the lower-warmer and fails to seep into the bladder. So the lower-warmer is distended. Water overflows, so water distention appears. The above is the normality or abnormality of the five kinds of metabolic liquids."

Commentary

This article makes an exposition about the fluids that are produced from water and grains, and their functions. The fluids of the body are sorted into two types. One is active fluids and the other is inactive fluids. With regard to their properties, the active fluids are relatively transparent and highly mobile. They mainly run at the body surface. They have the function of moistening the muscles and nourishing the skin. The inactive fluids are relatively thick and turbid. They are only slightly mobile. They mainly run in the viscera to moisten the bones, brain, marrow and orifices. However, on the whole, the active fluids and the inactive fluids can affect and transform each other. During the metabolic processes, these two kinds of fluids can be converted into sweat, urine, saliva, tears and dropsical water. They are called the five metabolic liquids.

Affected by the cold and heat of weather, and the thickness and thinness of clothes, sweat and urine can transform each other. That is to say, the five liquids can inter-transform. So edema could be treated by "diaphoresis and diuresis."

The article points out that if the *yin* and *yang* are out of equilibrium, such as from intemperate sexual activities, too many fluids will be lost, and the essential *yin* will become insufficient. After a long time, the symptom of painful back and loins will appear. If the four seas are obstructed, the triple-warmer fails to transport water, and the fluids fail to be transformed, causing water distention to appear. These descriptions are constructive to the "reason judgment and treatment determination" about painful back and loins and edema.

Annotation

[1] The five flavors of them rush into their own seas respectively: The liver and heart dominate the blood. So sour flavor and bitter flavor go to the sea of blood. The spleen dominates water and grains. So sweet flavor goes to the sea of water and grains. The lungs dominate the *qi*. So acrid flavor goes to the sea of *qi*. The kidneys dominate the marrow. Thus, salty flavor rushes to the sea of marrow.

[2] The triple-warmer transports the *qi*: The essential *qi* of foods is all transported and spread by the triple-warmer to the body. For example, the ancestral *qi* gathers at the upper-warmer; the nutritive *qi* comes from the middle-warmer; the defensive *qi* originates from the lower-warmer.

[3] The accumulated foam will induce pain: The fluids become coagulated and turn to foam as they receive cold.

[4] The spleen is the guard: The spleen dominates the muscles that protect the viscera.

[5] The kidneys govern the exterior: The kidneys govern storing the essence. They can steam and transform the fluids to nourish the skin. The kidneys are also where the defensive *qi* originates. The defensive *qi* can resist exogenous evils. So the kidneys dominate the exterior.

[6] The heart system: In this context, the vessels of the heart.

[7] Worms: Parasites in the intestines.

[8] If the *yin* and *yang* are uncoordinated: For example, intemperate sexual activities may create disharmony between the *yin* and *yang*.

2.15   Seventy-first Article

Dwelling of Evils · The Divine Pivot (*excerpt*)

Original article

Bo Gao said:

After the five cereals get into the stomach, the dregs, fluids and ancestral *qi* disperse in three different ways.[1] The ancestral *qi* accumulates in the chest and exits from the throat to penetrate the vessels of the heart, and control respiration there. The nutritive *qi* purifies fluids, rushes into the vessels, and turns into blood to nourish the four limbs and to irrigate the five *zang*-organs and six *fu*-organs regularly. The defensive *qi* is brave and runs swiftly. It first moves between the skin and muscles endlessly. The defensive *qi* flows in the *yang* aspect in the daytime, and runs in the *yin* aspect at night. Starting from the foot lesser-*yin* kidney channel, the defensive *qi* runs in the five *zang*-organs and six *fu*-organs at night.[2]

Commentary

This section mainly discusses the running routes, locations and major physiological functioning of the ancestral *qi*, nutritive *qi* and defensive *qi*. The ancestral *qi* accumulates in the chest. It has the function of running in the respiratory tract, controlling respiration, and penetrating the vessels of the heart. The nutritive *qi*, which runs in the vessels, is a component of the blood. It fills the five *zang*-organs and six *fu*-organs inside, and nourishes and fortifies the four limbs and bones outside. The defensive *qi* is a part of the *yang qi* of the body. It warms the muscles and skin, and it adjusts the opening and closing of the sweat pores.

Because the ancestral *qi* has the function of running in the respiratory tract, controlling respiration, penetrating the vessels of the heart, and pushing the blood, in clinical practice, when we observe symptoms due to *qi* deficiency manifested by low voice, disinclination to speak and shortness of breath, we think about the method of enriching the ancestral *qi*.

In fact, the nutritive *qi* and defensive *qi* are produced from the ancestral *qi*. So, if the ancestral *qi* is insufficient, deficiencies of the nutritive *qi* and defensive *qi* will occur.

If a patient has a shortage of the nutritive *qi* and defensive *qi*, especially the defensive *qi*, he will be susceptible to a cold, or he will have shortness of breath and perspire easily when moving about. Invigorating the ancestral *qi* may correct the problem.

Annotation

[1] The dregs, fluids and ancestral *qi* disperse in three different ways: The dregs are generated at the lower-warmer. The fluids are generated at the middle-warmer. The ancestral *qi* is generated at the upper-warmer.

[2] The defensive *qi* flows in the *yang* aspect in the daytime, and runs in the *yin* aspect at night. Starting from the foot lesser-*yin* kidney channel, the defensive *qi* runs in the five *zang*-organs and six *fu*-organs at night: The defensive *qi* runs in the *yang* aspect (i.e., superficial muscles) in the daytime, starting from the foot greater-*yang* bladder channel. It runs in the *yin* aspect, i.e., five *zang*-organs and six *fu*-organs at night, starting from the foot lesser-*yin* kidney channel.

2.16   Eighth Article

Root Spirit · The Divine Pivot

Original article

The Emperor asked: "Whether acupuncture would be effective is fundamentally based on the spirit of a patient. The blood, vessels, nutritive *qi*, and essence are stored by the five *zang*-organs. If one experiences excessive emotional frustration, the essence will be lost, and the soul will escape. Absent-mindedness will occur, and wisdom and thoughts will leave the body. Why does this happen? Is it the crime of the heaven? Is it the mistake of the patient? The virtue of the heaven and the benevolence of the earth produce men's spirit, essence, *yang* soul, *yin* soul, mind, idea, resolution, consideration, farsightedness, and wisdom. What about this?"

Uncle Qi answered: "The heaven bestows its virtue on people. The earth endows people with its benevolence. The virtue of the heaven descends, and the benevolence of the earth ascends so that people may live.[1] So, what is generated before birth is essence (sperm or ovum). Two essences wrestle, then the spirit is produced. The *yang* soul goes with the spirit.[2] The *yin* soul goes with the essence.[3] What learns and deals with things is mind. What is immature in the mind is idea. What is determined firmly is resolution. To think about this resolution over and over again is consideration. To ponder things from long distances and many angles is farsightedness. Dealing with all things with farsightedness is wisdom.

"So, when a man with wisdom cares for his life, he must obey the rules of seasons, and acclimatize to cold and heat. The man should appease joy and anger, and be satisfied with his residence. He should be moderate in the *yin* and *yang*, and adjust the rigidity and softness.[4] In this way, evils will not intrude, and one can live indefinitely.

"Therefore, fear and thought impair the spirit. The impaired spirit induces greater fear. Ceaseless seminal emission occurs.[5] When one's viscera are injured by sorrow, the *qi* of the viscera dries up, and his life is lost. Great joy makes the spirit escape and not be stored. Melancholy causes the *qi* to be blocked and stagnant. Rage causes one to be distracted and to lose self-control. Fear causes the spirit to dissipate and not be drawn back.

"Fear and thought of the heart impair the spirit. The impaired spirit induces greater fear, loss of self-control, haggardness, withered body hair and wizened color. The patient will die in the winter.[6] Unrestricted melancholy of the spleen damages the idea. The damaged idea makes depression, vexation, feeble limbs, withered body hair and wizened color. The patient will die in the spring.

"Sorrow of the liver injures the viscera and the *yang* soul. The injured *yang* soul causes madness, stupidity, huddling up and cramp when facing others, failure of sustenance of the ribs, withered body hair and wizened color. The patient will die in the autumn.

"Great joy of the lungs damages the *yin* soul. The damaged *yin* soul results in insanity, and behaving as if no one else were present. Dried-up skin, withered body hair and wizened color are also induced. The patient will die in the summer.

"Rage of the kidneys harms the resolution. The harmed resolution makes the patient forget what he has said, destroys the flexibility of his back, and causes withered body hair and wizened color. The patient will die in the late summer.

"Uncontrolled fear spoils the essence. The spoiled essence makes soft bones, atrophy, *qi* reversal and frequent seminal emissions. Therefore, the five *zang*-organs that store the essence should not be damaged, or the essence will not be conserved, and *yin* deficiency will occur. The *yin* deficiency makes the *qi* vacant. The vacant *qi* induces death.

"So an adept acupuncture doctor usually observes the state of the patient at length to know the existence or disappearance and gain or loss of the essence, spirit, *yang* soul, or *yin* soul. If the five *zang*-organs are injured, acupuncture will not be efficacious.

"The liver stores the blood. The *yang* soul dwells in the blood. Deficiency of the liver *qi* makes fear. Excess of the liver *qi* makes anger.

"The spleen stores the nutritive *qi*. The idea dwells in the nutritive *qi*. Deficiency of the spleen *qi* causes disabled limbs and uneasiness in the five *zang*-organs. Excess of the spleen *qi* makes abdominal distention, irregular menstruation, and impeded urine and stool.

"The heart stores the vessels. The spirit dwells in the vessels. Deficiency of the heart *qi* causes sorrow. Excess of the heart *qi* causes ceaseless laughing.

"The lungs store the *qi*. The *yin* soul dwells in the lungs. Deficiency of the lung *qi* causes nasal congestion and shortness of breath. Excess of the lung *qi* causes gasping, suffocated chest, and raising of the head for air.

"The kidneys store the resolution. The resolution dwells in the essence. Deficiency of the kidney *qi* causes *qi* reversal. Excess of the kidney *qi* causes distention and restlessness of the five *zang*-organs. Doctors should ascertain the level of illness of the five *zang*-organs to grasp the deficiency or excess of the *qi*, and adjust it meticulously."

Commentary

This article expounds the concepts of spirit, *yang* soul, *yin* soul, mind, idea, resolution, consideration, farsightedness, wisdom, etc. Their relationships with the five *zang*-organs are clearly explicated. The article points out that although human psychological and ideological activities are generally controlled by the mind, they are also separately governed by the five *zang*-organs. Excessively strong emotions can harm the *zang*-organs and induce disease. Conversely, the ill *zang*-organs can also induce abnormal emotional activities. The two issues interact as the cause and effect. This relationship is practically meaningful to the "syndrome identification and treatment determination", life care and anility resistance. In addition, some mental diseases will get worse, even to the point of causing death, when the seasons alter and the patients cannot adapt to the changes of seasons and climates. This is very common in clinical practice.

When the five *zang*-organs become unhealthy, psychological and emotional disorders appear. These symptoms can help us to analyze causes and determine treatments. For example, "deficiency of the liver *qi* makes fear, and excess of the liver *qi* makes anger." "Deficiency of the heart *qi* causes sorrow, and excess of the heart *qi* causes ceaseless laughing." These conditions are usually seen in clinical experience. What merits attention is that shortages of the spleen *qi* and kidney *qi* can make the five *zang*-organs restless. This idea is valuable in treating some chronic diseases and in the consolidation of effects. So, *The Discussion on the Spleen and Stomach*, an ancient medical masterpiece written by Li Dongyuan, provides the idea of "curing the spleen to pacify the five *zang*-organs."

At the end of the article, "doctors should ascertain the level of illness of the five *zang*-organs to grasp the deficiency or excess of the *qi*, and adjust it meticulously." They should strictly abide by this principle in treating the patient both by oral administration and by acupuncture.

Annotation

[1] The heaven bestows its virtue on people. The earth endows people with its benevolence. The virtue of the heaven descends, and the benevolence of the earth ascends so that people may live: The heaven provides climate, including sunshine, dew, rain, etc. The earth provides necessary conditions for living, including the five smells, five flavors, etc. The heaven and earth provide all living things with the necessary material conditions.

[2] The *yang* soul goes with the spirit: The *yang* soul is the *yang* part of the soul and pertains to the *yang*. The spirit pertains to the *yang* as well. The *yang* soul dominates a man's perception. The liver stores the *yang* soul.

[3] The *yin* soul goes with the essence: The *yin* soul is the *yin* part of the soul and pertains to the *yin*. The essence pertains to the *yin* as well. The *yin* soul dominates a man's movement. The lungs store the *yin* soul.

[4] Be moderate in the *yin* and *yang*, and adjust the rigidity and softness: Be moderate in sex.

[5] Ceaseless seminal emission occurs: Because fear damages the kidneys.

[6] The patient will die in the winter: Because water curbs fire, so a patient with heart disease will die in the winter. In the same way, the patient with the spleen disease will die in the spring; the patient with the liver disease will die in the autumn; the patient with the lung disease will die in the summer; the patient with the kidney disease will die in the late summer.

2.17   Forty-seventh Article

Root Zang-*Organs · The Divine Pivot* (*excerpt*)

Original article

The Emperor said to Uncle Qi:

Human blood, *qi*, essence and spirit are what supply existence and perfect life. The channels are where the *qi* and blood run in the ways of a *yin* and a *yang*. They are what moisten the tendons and bones, and what smooth the joints. The defensive *qi* is what warms the muscles, fills the skin, nourishes the muscular striae, and controls the opening and closing of the sweat pores.

The resolution and idea (i.e., the mind) are what govern the spirit, astringe the soul, adapt to cold and warmth, and appease joy and anger. Therefore, if the blood is harmonious, the channels will be unimpeded. The blood will run in the *yin* and *yang*.[1] The tendons and bones will be sinewy, and the joints will be flexible. If the defensive *qi* is harmonious, the muscles will move easily, the skin will be smooth, and the muscular striae will be compact.

If the resolution and idea (i.e., mind) are harmonious, the brain will be shrewd, and the *yang* soul and *yin* soul will not be detached. Neither penitence nor anger will arise, and the five *zang*-organs will not be attacked by evils. If the cold and warmth are harmonious, the six *fu*-organs will transform grains. Wind evil will not attack from outside, and numbness will not appear from within. The channels will be free, and the limbs will be in comfort. These are normal conditions to healthy people. The five *zang*-organs are what store the essence, spirit, blood, *qi*, *yang* soul and *yin* soul. The six *fu*-organs are what transform water and grains and move fluids. All these functions of the viscera are innate endowments. All people, whether stupid or clever, have these without reference to their stupidity or cleverness.

Commentary

This section summarizes the important roles of the blood, *qi*, spirit, essence, channels, defensive *qi*, and mind. It points out that, though the blood, *qi*, spirit, essence, defensive *qi*, soul, channels, etc., originate from the essential *qi* of the five *zang*-organs and six *fu*-organs, they play the role of protecting the *zang-fu* organs. So, if the functions of the viscera are coordinated, one will be healthy, or one will not. The article underlines that making the blood smooth, adjusting the emotions, acclimatizing to changes of climate, etc., are important to assure the normal functioning of the viscera. This discussion emphasizes that a man is an organic entity and that humans are closely related to the natural circumstances.

Annotation
[1] The blood will run in the *yin* and *yang*: i.e., the exterior and interior of the body.

Chapter Three
Theory of Channels and Network-Channels

The theory of channels and network-channels covers research into the physiological functioning and pathogenic changes of the system of channels and network-channels in man. It is an important part of the theoretical system of TCM. The primary functions of channels and network-channels are running the *qi* and blood of the whole body, linking the *zang-fu* organs and limbs, and connecting the upper part, lower part, interior, and exterior. Therefore, the channels and network-channels interconnect all parts of the body into one organic entity.

The theory of channels and network-channels is highly significant to physiology and pathology. It also plays a certain directive role in various clinical subjects, especially to acupuncture, which uses this theory as its rationale.

The contents of this theory comprise two parts, i.e., the channels and the network-channels. Channels are the major concern.

The channels are the main trunks of the networks of body channels and network-channels. The channels can be divided into two groups. The first group is the twelve main channels, including the corresponding six *yang* channels and six *yin* channels: the hand greater-*yin* lung channel, hand cold-*yin* pericardium channel, hand lesser-*yin* heart channel, hand greater-*yang* small-intestine channel, hand lesser-*yang* triple-warmer channel, hand bright-*yang* large-intestine channel, foot bright-*yang* stomach channel, foot lesser-*yang* gallbladder channel, foot greater-*yang* bladder channel, foot lesser-*yin* kidney channel, foot cold-*yin* liver channel, and foot greater-*yin* spleen channel.

The twelve main channels are named according to the *zang*-organ and *fu*-organ, the foot and hand, and the *yin* and *yang* of the front, middle, and back locations. When a man stands naturally, the front of the body is *yin*, and the back of the body is *yang*. The inner faces of the limbs are *yin*, and the outer faces of the limbs are *yang*.

The second group is eight peculiar channels, i.e., the controlling channel, governing channel, penetrating channel, girdling channel, *yin*-linking channel, *yang*-linking channel, *yin*-springing channel, and *yang*-springing channel.

The network-channels are thinner than the channels and are the branches of the networks of human channels and network-channels. They crisscross the body and are usually separated into three types. The first type is the fifteen branched network-channels. The second is the floating network-channels, which can be seen running in the shallow parts. The third is the grandchild network-channels, which are the thinnest, most widespread, and are innumerable. The twelve main channels, the governing channel, and the controlling channel each branch into a network-channel.

Adding the big network-channel of the spleen, they constitute the fifteen branched network-channels, which can intensify the links of the external channels and internal channels, and can help communication of the *qi* at the abdomen, back, and flanks.

In addition, there exist twelve channel divergences, twelve channel sinews, and twelve skin regions. Every main channel diverges into another channel at the region around the knee or elbow. Every diverged channel runs deeply into the body cavity, connects with concerned *zang-fu* organs, and then moves out to the shallow part of the head or neck. So, there are twelve channel divergences in all, which can intensify the connection of the *zang-fu* organs to every couple of interior-exterior channels. Every main channel has a sinew that starts from the distal end of a limb and goes to the head and body. Each sinew runs superficially to bind the bones, and smooth the movements of the joints. So they are called the twelve channel sinews.

Each main channel has its own access area on the covering skin. These areas are called the twelve skin regions. Because the routes of the twelve channel sinews and the locations of the twelve skin regions are approximately identical to the superficial locations of the twelve main channels, they are named according to the twelve main channels; they also pertain to the field of the twelve main channels.

In order to assist the student, illustrations of the systematic structure of the channels and network-channels have been sought and are included in this volume.

The following lists show the channels and network-channels in their logical order.

Systematic Structure of Channels and Network-Channels

Lists of Channels and Network-Channels
1. Channels
1.1   Twelve Main Channels
hand bright-*yang* large-intestine channel (LI channel)
hand lesser-*yang* triple – warmer channel (TW channel)
hand greater-*yang* small-intestine channel (SI channel)
hand lesser-*yin* heart channel (HT channel)
hand cold-*yin* pericardium channel (PC channel)
hand greater-*yin* lung channel (LU channel)
foot bright-*yang* stomach channel (ST channel)
foot lesser-*yang* gallbladder channel (GB channel)
foot greater-*yang* bladder channel (BL channel)
foot lesser-*yin* kidney channel (KI channel)

foot cold-*yin* liver channel (LV channel)
foot greater-*yin* spleen channel (SP channel)

1.2   Eight Peculiar Channels
controlling channel (CT channel)
governing channel (GV channel)
penetrating channel (PT channel)
girdling channel (GD channel)
yin-linking channel (YIL channel)
yang-linking channel (YAL channel)
yin-springing channel (YIS channel)
yang-springing channel (YAS channel)

1.3   Affiliated Structures of Channels
twelve channel divergences
twelve channel sinews
twelve skin regions

2. Network-Channels
fifteen branched network-channels
floating network-channels
grandchild network-channels

3.1   Tenth Article

Channels · The Divine Pivot (excerpt)

3.1.1   Original article

Lei Gong[1] asked the Emperor: "*The Commandment of Teaching*[2] says: All rules of needling begin from the channels. Doctors seek for their routes and measure the lengths of the channels that connect with the five *zang*-organs inside, and link up with the six *fu*-organs outside. Please tell me all the details."

The Emperor answered: "Every life begins as the mixed essences of the parents. The brains are produced after the essences are mixed. The bones support the body. The channels irrigate the body. The tendons make the body strong. The muscles protect the body like walls. The skin becomes more firm and the body hair grows. After grains enter the stomach, the ways of the channels become free; then the *qi* and blood run in them."

Lei Gong asked: "Please tell me the functions of the channels when they were produced."

The Emperor answered: "The channels can determine death and life, deal with the hundred different diseases, and adjust deficiency and excess. Doctors must be proficient in knowledge of the channels."

Commentary

This article talks about the value of the theory of channels and network-channels in diagnosis and treatment, and stresses the importance of mastering this theory. It has been proved that when a disease occurs, it is transferred from the exterior to the interior or from the interior to the exterior, with the channels as the usual transmission routes. The symptoms that are presented during a transmission can be seen on the corresponding body surface along the disordered channels. The system of channels and network-channels reflects symptoms reliably.

With this information, we can determine the place, property, and prognosis of a disease. This idea is one of the significant theories for clinical syndrome identification, i.e., the syndrome identification of channels and network-channels. When doctors choose treatment, this theory is suitable for use in all clinical subjects. Specifically, the therapeutic principle of "selecting acupuncture points along channels" in acupuncture is wholly based on the theory of channels and network-channels. Moreover, the theory of channel tropism in materia medica of TCM is under the guidance of the theory of channels and network-channels. Because this theory is so important, all medical masters of past times paid lavish attention to it. As a master said: "A doctor who does not know the channels is like a person who walks in the night without a candle."

Annotation
[1] Lei Gong: The youngest minister of the Yellow Emperor.
[2] *The Commandment of Teaching*: The forty-eighth article in *The Divine Pivot*.

3.1.2   Original article

"The hand greater-*yin* lung channel[1] starts[2] from the middle-warmer, descends[2] to link[2] up with the large intestine, returns[2] and moves along[2] the mouths of the stomach,[3] ascends[2] across the diaphragm, pertains[2] to the lung, traverses[2] the lung system,[4] gets out[2] of the armpit, descends along the upper arm and passes[2] before the hand cold-*yin* pericardium channel,[5] descends the elbow, moves along the back edge of the radius[6] at the inner face of the forearm,[7] gets into[2] the pulse spot of the wrist, descends to the fish-abdomen-style muscles,[8] moves along the front edge of the fish-abdomen-style muscles, and gets out[2] of the end of the thumb. The channel's branch goes directly to the front margin of the outer face of the forefinger from above the wrist, and gets out of its end.[9]

"So, once the lung channel has been disordered, the patient suffers from distention and fullness of the lungs, gasping, coughing, and has pain in the supraclavicular fossae, and even to the point of clasping the arms and having blurred vision during a severe cough. The disease is called *qi* reversal of the arm.[10] Therefore, the channel dominates diseases due to disorders of the lungs. The symptoms are coughing, rough gasping, vexation, a full chest, pains along the front edges of the inner faces of the upper arms and forearms, and a hot sensation in the centers of the palms.

"If the *qi* of the lung channel is exuberant and excessive, the patient will have painful shoulders and back due to wind and cold, sweating, wind stroke, and frequent and scant urine. If its *qi* is deficient, the patient will have painful shoulders and back due to cold, shortness of breath, and urine of changed color. To treat such diseases, drain what is excessive, and supplement what is deficient. Needle fast to what has heat, retain needles to what has cold,[11] and use moxibustion to what shows sinking. If a disease is due to neither excess nor deficiency of other channels, select the lung channel itself.[12] If the *qi* of the channel is excessive, the wrist pulse will be three times larger than the neck pulse.[13] If the *qi* is deficient, the wrist pulse will be smaller than the neck pulse.

"The hand bright-*yang* large-intestine channel[14] starts from the end of the forefinger, moves along the front edge of the forefinger, gets out of the *hegu point between the first metacarpal bone and the second metacarpal bone, ascends and gets into the wrist pit between the two tendons,*[15] moves a-long the front edge of the forearm, gets into the outer face of the elbow, as-cends the front edge of the outer face of the upper arm, ascends the shoulder, gets out of the front edge of the crossing point of the clavicle and scapula, as-cends and gets out of the *dazhui* point under the pillar bone,[16] descends to get into the supraclavicular fossa, links up with the lung, descends across the di-aphragm, and pertains to the large-intestine. Its branch ascends from the supraclavicular fossa to the neck and penetrates the cheek, gets into the lower gums, returns and gets out to clamp the mouth,[17] and crosses at the philtrum. The left line runs to the right, and the right line runs to the left. The branch ascends and clamps the nostril.

"So, once the large-intestine channel has been disordered, the patient suffers from painful teeth and swollen neck. The channel dominates diseases due to disorders of the fluids.[18] These diseases are characterized by yellow eyes, a dry mouth, nasal congestion and bleeding, a swollen throat, pains at the fronts of the shoulders and at the forearms, and painful and disabled thumbs and forefingers.

"If the *qi* of the large-intestine channel is excessive, the area where its channel runs through will be hot and swollen. If its *qi* is deficient, one will shudder and find it difficult to keep warm. To treat such diseases, drain what is excessive, and supplement what is deficient. Needle fast to what shows heat, retain needles to what has cold, and use moxibustion to what shows sinking. If a disease is due to neither excess nor deficiency of other channels, select the large-intestine channel itself. If its *qi* is excessive, the neck pulse will be three times larger than the wrist pulse. If its *qi* is deficient, the neck pulse will be smaller than the wrist pulse.

"The foot bright-*yang* stomach channel[19] starts from the sinking place of the nose bridge, wraps the *jing-ming* point[20] where the foot greater-*yang* bladder channel originates, descends beside the nose, gets into the upper gums, returns out and goes around the lips, descends to cross at the *chengjiang* point,[21] recedes to move along the lower edge of the cheek, gets out of the *daying* point,[22] moves along the *jiache* point,[23] ascends before the ear, passes the *shangguan* point,[24] moves along the edge of hair, and reaches the forehead.

"A branch descends to the *renying* point from the front of the *daying* point, moves along the throat, gets into the supraclavicular fossa, descends across the diaphragm, pertains to the stomach, and links up with the spleen. The direct line descends the inner side of the breast from the supraclavicular fossa, descends to clamp the umbilicus, and gets into the *qichong* point.[25]

"Another branch starts from the lower mouth of the stomach, descends along the inside of the abdomen, reaches the *qichong* point to merge with the foregoing line, descends the *biguan* point,[26] reaches the *futu* point,[27] descends to the patella, descends along the front edge of the outer side of the tibia, descends the instep, gets into the outer edge beside the second toenail.

"Its branch diverges at a point, which is three thumb-widths below the knee, and descends to get into the outer edge beside the middle toenail.

"Its another branch diverges at the instep, gets into the big toe and gets out of its end.

"So, once the stomach channel has been disordered, the patient shivers with cold and is prone to moan and yawn frequently, and his forehead is black. When the disease is coming on, the patient dislikes being around people and dislikes fire. He becomes frightened suddenly when hearing wood sounds. His heart is agitated. He stays alone, with the door and windows closed, even desiring to climb a high place to sing, and wanting to cast off his clothes to run. The intestines and stomach thunder, and the abdomen is distended. This disease is called *qi* reversal of the tibia.[28]

"Therefore, the channel dominates diseases due to disorders of the blood.[29] These disorders are characterized by mania, warm malaria, sweating,[30] nasal congestion and bleeding, an awry mouth, small blisters on the lips, swollen neck and throat, abdomen large with edema, and swollen and painful knees and patellae. Painful lines from the breasts to the *qichong* points, thighs, *futu* points, outer sides of the tibias, and insteps, and disabled middle toes are also presented.

"If the *qi* of the stomach channel is excessive, the front of the body will be hot all over. If the *qi* is surplus in the stomach, the patient will digest grains quickly and will usually be hungry, and his urine will be darkish. If its *qi* is deficient, the front of the body will be chilly, and the stomach will be cold, distended and full. To treat such diseases, drain what is excessive, and supplement what is deficient. Needle fast to what has heat, retain needles to what has cold, and use moxibustion to what shows sinking. If a disease is due to neither excess nor deficiency of other channels, select the stomach channel itself. If its *qi* is excessive, the neck pulse will be three times larger than the wrist pulse. If its *qi* is deficient, the neck pulse will be smaller than the wrist pulse.

"The foot greater-*yin* spleen channel[31] starts from the end of the big toe, moves along the inner edge of the white muscles of the foot, goes to the back of the nut-like bone,[32] ascends the front edge of the medial malleolus, ascends the inner side of the shank, moves along the back of the tibia, crosses the foot cold-*yin* liver channel and goes before it, ascends the front edge of the inner face of the knee and thigh, gets into the abdomen, pertains to the spleen, links up with the stomach, ascends across the diaphragm, clamps the throat, connects with the tongue root, and spreads under the tongue. Its branch diverges from the stomach to ascend across the diaphragm, and rushes into the heart.

"So, once the spleen channel has been disordered, the patient suffers from stiff tongue root, vomiting after eating, painful stomach duct, abdominal distention, and a tendency to hiccup. He feels quite relaxed after discharging feces and gas, and his body is unwieldy. Therefore, the channel dominates diseases due to disorders of the spleen. The symptoms are painful tongue root, inability to shake the body, difficult swallowing, vexation, acute pains under the heart, loose stool, conglomeration, diarrhea, obstruction of urine, jaundice, inability to lie,[33] narrow standing, swollen and cold inner faces of the knees and thighs, and disabled big toes.

"To treat such diseases, drain what is excessive, and supplement what is deficient. Needle fast to what has heat, retain needles to what has cold, and use moxibustion to what shows sinking. If a disease is due to neither excess nor deficiency of other channels, select the spleen channel itself. If its *qi* is excessive, the wrist pulse will be three times larger than the neck pulse. If its *qi* is deficient, the wrist pulse will be smaller than the neck pulse.

"The hand lesser-*yin* heart channel[34] starts from the inside of the heart, gets out and connects with the heart system,[35] descends across the diaphragm, and links up with the small-intestine.

"Its branch ascends from the heart system, clamps the throat, and connects with the eye system.[36]

"Its direct line ascends the lung from the heart system, descends to get out of the armpit, descends along the back edge of the inner face of the upper arm running after the hand greater-*yin* lung channel and hand cold-*yin* pericardium channel, descends the inner side of the elbow, moves along the back edge of the inner face of the forearm, reaches the end of the ulnar head above the palm, gets into the back edge of the palm, moves along the inner face of the little finger, and gets out of its end.

"So, once the heart channel has been disordered, the patient suffers from a dry throat, a painful heart, and constant thirst. This disease is called *qi* reversal of the arm. Therefore, the channel dominates diseases due to disorders of the heart. These are presented as yellow eyes, painful rib-sides, painful and cold back edges of the inner faces of the upper-arms and forearms, and hot and painful centers of the palms.

"To treat such diseases, drain what is excessive, and supplement what is deficient. Needle fast to what has heat, retain needles to what has cold, and use moxibustion to what shows sinking. If a disease is due to neither excess nor deficiency of other channels, select the heart channel itself. If its *qi* is excessive, the wrist pulse will be twice as large as the neck pulse. If its *qi* is deficient, the wrist pulse will be smaller than the neck pulse.

"The hand greater-*yang* small-intestine channel[37] starts from the end of the little finger, moves along the back edge of the back of hand, ascends the wrist, gets out of the ulnar process above the wrist, ascends directly along the back edge of the ulna, gets out between the two bones[38] at the outer face of the elbow, ascends along the back edge of the outer face of upper arm, gets out of the shoulder joint, gets around the scapula, crosses the governing channel at the *dazhui* point above the shoulder, gets into the supraclavicular fossa, links up with the heart, moves down along the esophagus, descends across the diaphragm, reaches the stomach, and pertains to the small-intestine.

"A branch moves upward along the neck from the supraclavicular fossa, ascends the cheek, arrives at the outer canthus, and recedes into the ear.

"Another branch diverges at the cheek, ascends below the eye, reaches the nose, arrives at the inner canthus, and connects with the cheekbone on a diagonal.

"So, once the small-intestine channel has been disordered, the patient suffers from a painful throat, a swollen chin, inability to turn the head, seemingly plucked shoulders, and seemingly broken upper arms. Therefore, the small-intestine channel dominates diseases due to disorders of the fluids.[39] The presented symptoms are deafness, yellow eyes, swollen cheeks, and painful neck, chin and shoulders, also aching in the back edges of the outer faces of the upper-arms, elbows and forearms.

"To treat such diseases, drain what is excessive, and supplement what is deficient. Needle fast to what has heat, retain needles to what has cold, and use moxibustion to what shows sinking. If a disease is due to neither excess nor deficiency of other channels, select the small-intestine channel itself. If its *qi* is excessive, the neck pulse will be twice as large as the wrist pulse. If its *qi* is deficient, the neck pulse will be smaller than the wrist pulse.

"The foot greater-*yang* bladder channel[40] starts from the inner canthus, ascends the forehead, and crosses the governing channel at the vertex. Its branch reaches the upper corner of the ear from the vertex. Its straight line gets in to connect with the brain from the vertex, returns out, diverges and descends the neck, moves along the inner side beside the scapula, clamps the spine, reaches the loin, gets in through the muscles beside the spine, links up with the kidney, and pertains to the bladder.

"A branch descends from the loin, clamps the spine, penetrates the hip, and gets into the back of the knee.

"Another branch penetrates downward the inner edge of the scapula, clamps the side of the spine, goes through the hip joint, moves along the outer edge of the hip, descends the outer edge of the back face of the thigh, merges at the back of the knee, descends and penetrates the calf, gets out behind the lateral malleolus, reaches the outer edge beside the little toenail along the process of the fifth metatarsal bone.

"So, once the bladder channel has been disordered, the patient suffers from *qi*-surging headache,[41] seemingly fallen eyes, seemingly plucked neck, painful spine, seemingly broken waist, inability to flex the hips, and seemingly locked knees and broken calves. The disease is called *qi* reversal of the ankle. Therefore, the channel dominates diseases due to disorders of the tendons.[42] The symptoms presented are hemorrhoids, malaria, mania, madness, painful vertex and neck, yellow eyes, shedding tears, nasal congestion and bleeding, painful neck, back, loins, sacrum, backs of the knees, calves and feet, and disabled little toes.

"To treat such diseases, drain what is excessive, and supplement what is deficient. Needle fast to what has heat, retain needles to what has cold, and use moxibustion to what shows sinking. If a disease is due to neither excess nor deficiency of other channels, select the bladder channel itself. If its *qi* is excessive, the neck pulse will be twice as large as the wrist pulse. If its *qi* is deficient, the neck pulse will be smaller than the wrist pulse.

"The foot lesser-*yin* kidney channel[43] starts from the bottom of the little toe, runs diagonally to the center of the sole, gets out under the *rangu* point,[44] moves along the back of the medial malleolus, gets into the heel, ascends the inner face of the shank, gets out of the inner face of the knee, ascends the back edge of the inner face of the thigh, penetrates the spine, pertains to the kidney, and links up with the bladder. Its straight line penetrates upward across the liver and diaphragm, gets into the lung, moves along the throat, and clamps the root of the tongue. Its branch gets out of the lung, connects with the heart, and rushes into the chest.

"So, once the kidney channel has been disordered, the patient suffers from hunger without appetite, face dark like burnt wood, coughing and spitting with blood, and gasping with hoarse and whimpering sounds. He wants to stand up rather than sitting. His sight is blurred to the point of being cloudy. He feels his heart pendent as if in hunger. The patient is prone to be frightened, when the *qi* is insufficient. He is highly fearful as if someone will arrest him. The disease is called *qi* reversal of the bone.[45]

"Therefore, the channel dominates diseases due to disorders of the kidneys. These are characterized by hot mouth, dry tongue, swollen pharynx, *qi* ascent,[46] dry and painful larynx, vexation, painful heart, jaundice, intestinal flux,[47] painful spine and back edges of the inner faces of the thighs, atrophy, *qi* reversal, somnolence, and hot and painful soles.

"To treat such diseases, drain what is excessive, and supplement what is deficient. Needle fast to what has heat, retain needles to what has cold, and use moxibustion to what shows sinking. If a disease is due to neither excess nor deficiency of other channels, select the kidney channel itself. Moxibustion could enhance the patient's appetite, and rich flavors can promote the growth of muscles. The patient should loosen his laces, wear the hair down, and walk leisurely holding a big cane and wearing heavy shoes.[48] If its *qi* is excessive, the wrist pulse will be twice as large as the neck pulse. If its *qi* is deficient, the wrist pulse will be smaller than the neck pulse.

"The hand cold-*yin* pericardium channel[49] starts from the chest, gets out and pertains to the pericardium, descends across the diaphragm, and connects with the three warmers, in order.[50]

"A branch moves along the chest, gets out of the rib-side three thumb-widths under the armpit, ascends to reach the armpit, moves along the inner face of the upper arm running between the hand greater-*yin* lung channel and hand lesser-*yin* heart channel, gets into the elbow, descends the forearm running between the two tendons, gets into the palm, moves along the middle finger, and gets out of its end.

"Another branch diverges at the palm, moves along the third finger, and gets out of its end.

"So, once the pericardium channel has been disordered, the patient suffers from hot palmar centers, spasmodic arms and elbows, swollen armpits, even propped-full chest and rib-sides, great throbbing of the heart, a red face, yellow eyes, and endless joyful laughing. Therefore, the channel dominates diseases due to disorders of the vessels.[51] These are characterized by vexation, painful heart, hot centers of the palms.

"To treat such diseases, drain what is excessive, and supplement what is deficient. Needle fast to what has heat, retain needles to what has cold, and use moxibustion to what shows sinking. If a disease is due to neither excess nor deficiency of other channels, select the pericardium channel itself. If its *qi* is excessive, the wrist pulse will be as large as the neck pulse. If its *qi* is deficient, the wrist pulse will be smaller than the neck pulse.

"The hand lesser-*yang* triple-warmer channel[52] starts from the end of the third finger, ascends to get out of the two fingers,[53] moves along the outer face of the hand, gets out between the two bones[54] at the outer face of the forearm, ascends to penetrate the elbow, moves along the outer face of the upper arm, mounts the shoulder, crosses the foot lesser-*yang* gallbladder channel and runs after it, gets into the supraclavicular fossa, spreads in the chest, connects with the pericardium, descends across the diaphragm, and pertains to the triple-warmer.

"A branch ascends from the chest to get out of the supraclavicular fossa, ascends the neck, moves directly upward behind the ear, gets out of the upper corner of the ear, curves to descend the cheek, and reaches the region under the eye socket.

"Another branch gets into the ear from the back of the ear, gets out and runs before the ear, passes before the *shangguan* point,[55] crosses the former line at the cheek, and reaches the outer canthus.

"So, once the triple-warmer has been disordered, the patient suffers from deafness, or muffled hearing, a swollen pharynx, and a numb larynx. Therefore, the channel dominates diseases due to disorders of the *qi*.[56] These are marked by sweating, painful canthi, and aching cheeks. Painful backs of the ears and shoulders, and aching outer faces of the upper arms and elbows and forearms are also presented. The third fingers are disabled.

"To treat such diseases, drain what is excessive, and supplement what is deficient. Needle fast to what has heat, retain needles to what has cold, and use moxibustion to what shows sinking. If a disease is due to neither excess nor deficiency of other channels, select the triple-warmer itself. If its *qi* is excessive, the neck pulse will be as large as the wrist pulse. If its *qi* is deficient, the neck pulse will be smaller than the wrist pulse.

"The foot lesser-*yang* gallbladder channel[57] starts from the outer canthus, ascends to reach the corner of the forehead, descends to the back of the ear, moves along the neck before the hand lesser-*yang* triple-warmer channel, reaches the shoulder, recedes to cross the hand lesser-*yang* channel and runs after it, and gets into the supraclavicular fossa.

"A branch gets into the ear from the back of the ear, gets out and runs before the ear, and reaches the region behind the outer canthus.

"Another branch diverges at the outer canthus, descends the *daying* point, merges with the hand lesser-*yang* channel to reach the region under the eye socket, descends through the *jiache* point, descends the neck to merge with the former line at the supraclavicular fossa, descends the chest, penetrates across the diaphragm, links up with the liver, pertains to the gall-bladder, moves along the inside of the rib-side, gets out of the *qichong* point, gets around the pubic region, and traverses into the thigh pivot.

"Its straight line descends the armpit from the supraclavicular fossa, moves along the flank of the chest, goes through the hypochondrium, descends to merge at the thigh pivot, descends along the outer face of the thigh, gets out of the outer side of the knee, descends before the fibula, descends directly to the lower end of the fibula, descends to get out before the lateral malleolus, moves along the instep, and gets into the outer edge beside the third toenail. Another branch diverges at the instep, gets into the big toe along the fissure between the first and second metatarsal bones, gets out of its end, returns and penetrates the toenail, and gets out of the hair region behind its toenail.

"So, once the gallbladder channel has been disordered, the patient suffers from a bitter taste in the mouth, frequent sighing, painful heart and rib-sides, inability to turn the body, possibly even feeling that his face is slightly dust-covered,[58] absence of sheen and gloss of the body, abnormally hot outer faces of the legs. The disease is called *qi* reversal of *yang*.[59] Therefore, the channel dominates diseases due to disorders of the bones.[60] The symptoms are headache, painful chin and outer canthi, swollen and painful supraclavicular fossae, swollen armpits, sabre-shaped and connecting pear-shaped scrofula,[61] sweating, shuddering with cold, malaria, and painful chest flanks and rib-sides. The painful outer faces of the thighs and knees and fibulas, and aching front parts of the lateral malleoli are also presented. All concerned joints are painful and the third toes are disabled.

"To treat such diseases, drain what is excessive, and supplement what is deficient. Needle fast to what has heat, retain needles to what has cold, and use moxibustion to what shows sinking. If a disease is due to neither excess nor deficiency of other channels, select the gallbladder channel itself. If its *qi* is excessive, the neck pulse will be as large as the wrist pulse. If its *qi* is deficient, the neck pulse will be smaller than the wrist pulse.

"The foot cold-*yin* liver channel[62] starts from the hair-growing region of the great toe, ascends along the upper edge of the instep, passes before the medial malleolus a thumb-width away, crosses the foot greater-*yin* spleen channel and runs after it when being eight thumb-widths above the malleolus, ascends the inner side of the knee, moves along the inner face of the thigh, gets into the pubes, gets around the genitals, reaches the lower abdomen, clamps the stomach, pertains to the liver, links up with the gallbladder, ascends to penetrate across the diaphragm, spreads at the rib-side, moves along the back of the throat, ascends to get into the palate, connects with the eye system, ascends to get out of the forehead, and meets the governing channel at the vertex.

"A branch descends the inner side of the cheek from the eye system, and gets around the inside of the lips.

"Another branch diverges again from the liver, penetrates across the diaphragm, ascends to rush into the lung.

"So, once the liver channel has been disordered, the patient suffers from painful waist, inability to bend forward and backward, male prominent hernia,[63] or female swollen lower abdomen, even a dry throat, and the feeling of dust-covered face with loss of color. Therefore, the channel dominates diseases due to disorders of the liver. These are characterized by full chest, vomiting, diarrhea containing undigested foods, fox hernia,[64] bedwetting, and obstruction of urine.

"To treat such diseases, drain what is excessive, and supplement what is deficient. Needle fast to what has heat, retain needles to what has cold, and use moxibustion to what shows sinking. If a disease is due to neither excess nor deficiency of other channels, select the liver channel itself. If its *qi* is excessive, the wrist pulse will be as large as the neck pulse. If its *qi* is deficient, the wrist pulse will be smaller than the neck pulse."

Commentary

The above twelve segments separately describe the running routes of the twelve main channels and their dominated diseases and symptoms. The therapeutic principles of acupuncture applied to the diseases and signs of deficiency, excess, cold, heat, and neither excess nor deficiency, are the major topics of the theory of channels and network-channels. The twelve main channels are the main passages for the running of the *qi* and blood. The channels have direct connections with the *zang-fu* organs. The *yin* channels pertain to the *zang*-organs and link up with the *fu*-organs. The *yang* channels pertain to the *fu*-organs and link up with the *zang*-organs. The correspondences of interior-exterior of the *zang-fu* organs, and the links of all other organs entirely rely on the twelve main channels for fulfillment.

So we say that the twelve channels pertain to the *zang-fu* organs inside and connect with the limbs outside. In clinical practice, the theory of channels and network-channels and the theory of *zang*-organs and manifestations should be combined. In this way, physicians can beneficially open their thoughts and widen their understanding of therapeutic methods in analyzing pathology and diagnosing and curing diseases.

The major diseases of a main channel do not go beyond the disorders of where the channel passes and of the pertained and linked *zang*-organ and *fu*-organ. Take, for example, the hand greater-*yin* lung channel. The symptoms of painful supraclavicular fossae, even dizziness with clasping of the hands, painful front edges of the inner faces of the arms, and hot palmar centers, are the disorders of where the lung channel passes. These pathogenic manifestations are the basis for clinical syndrome identifications. In addition, we exclusively take the running route of a channel as a major reference to diagnosis, such as the syndrome identification of the six channels to headache, the discriminations of the numbness of the fingers, the places of the numb limbs, etc. This kind of syndrome identification in diagnostics is generally called syndrome identification of channels and network-channels.

Annotation

[1] The hand greater-*yin* lung channel: It is abbreviated as the LU channel. A person's *qi* and blood start to run from this channel, then run to the large-intestine channel, stomach channel, spleen channel, heart channel, small-intestine channel, bladder channel, kidney channel, pericardium channel, triple-warmer channel, gallbladder channel, and liver channel, in that order. When the *qi* and blood return to the lung channel from the liver channel, another circulation begins.

[2] Start, link, pertain, return, move along, traverse, pass, ascend, descend, get out and get in: These verbs are used to describe the running routes of the channels. The beginning of the running route of a channel is the start. When a channel connects with its corresponding *zang*-organ or *fu*-organ, it is said to link. When a channel connects with its pertained *zang*-organ or *fu*-organ, it is said to pertain. When a channel goes ahead and then returns back, it is said to return. When a channel goes along in a certain direction, it is said to move along. Moving horizontally is traversing. Passing in the vicinity of another channel is passing. Going from the lower part to the upper part is ascending. Going from the upper part to the lower part is descending. Running from the deep part to the shallow part is getting out. Running from the exterior to the interior is getting in.

[3] The mouths of the stomach: Both the upper and lower mouths of the stomach.

[4] The lung system: Refers to the trachea, throat and other tissues that connect with the lungs.

[5] Before the hand cold-*yin* pericardium channel: When a man stands naturally, the radial side is the front; so the lung channel runs before the cold-*yin* pericardium channel, which runs between

the radius and ulna. The cold-*yin* pericardium channel runs before the hand lesser-*yin* heart channel, which is located on the ulnar side.

[6] The back edge of the radius: When a man stands naturally, the radial side is usually regarded as the front side, and the ulnar side is usually regarded as the back side.

[7] The inner face of the forearm: When a man stands naturally, the faces of the arms pressing the body are usually regarded as the inner faces. The opposite sides are outer faces.

[8] The fish-abdomen-style muscles: The muscles above the thumb at the palm bulge like the fish's belly.

[9] And gets out of its end: In order to connect with the hand bright-*yang* large-intestine channel.

[10] The disease is called *qi* reversal of the arm: The above-mentioned symptoms are due to reversal and disorder of the arm *qi*.

[11] Needle fast to what has heat, retain needles to what has cold: Needle fast in a heat case. Let needles stay at certain points for a designated period of time in order to enhance the effect in a cold case.

[12] When a disease is due to neither excess nor deficiency of other channels, select the lung channel itself: If the lung channel contracts evils itself without being affected by other excessive or deficient channels, we should drain or supplement the lung channel itself.

[13] The neck pulse: Also known as the *renying* pulse, i.e., ST-9 who; an important place for pulse-taking, where the carotid pulsates beside the Adam's apple.

[14] The hand bright-*yang* large-intestine channel: Abbreviated as the LI channel.

[15] The two tendons: The pollical short-stretch tendon and the pollical long-stretch tendon.

[16] The *dazhui* point under the pillar bone: The seventh cervical vertebra is prominent, so it is called the pillar bone. The *dazhui* point (GV-14 who, i.e., Great Hammer) pertaining to the governing channel is under the spinal process of the seventh cervical vertebra. Many *yang* channels meet at the *dazhui* point.

[17] Clamp the mouth: When two lines of a channel run through both sides of the same anatomical structure, it is called clamping.

[18] Diseases due to disorders of the fluids: The large-intestine transmits water and grains, and transforms essential materials, so the large-intestine dominates diseases due to disorders of the fluids. Furthermore, the large-intestine and lungs stand in exterior-interior, and the lungs dominate the *qi* that governs the transformations of the fluids. So both diarrhea and constipation of the large-intestine are due to disorders of the fluids.

[19] The foot bright-*yang* stomach channel: Abbreviated as the ST channel.

[20] The *jing-ming* point: BL-1, i.e., Bright Essence; the inner canthus where the foot greater-*yang* bladder channel originates.

[21] The *chengjiang* point: Also known as CV-24 who, i.e., Sauce Receptacle; the center of the groove under the mouth, pertaining to the controlling channel.

[22] The *daying* point: ST-5 who, i.e., Great Reception; the front edge of the spot to which the biting muscles adhere. When one closes his mouth and bulges the cheeks with air, a depression will appear at the lower jaw. Select the *daying* point at the lower end of the depression.

[23] The *jiache* point: ST-6 who, i.e., Cheek Carriage; the highest point of the biting muscles when one masticates, about a transverse-finger away from the corner of the lower jaw.

[24] The *shangguan* point: GB-3 who, i.e., Upper Gate; a little above the upper edge of the cheekbone, in the depression, about a thumb-width away from the front edge of the auricle.

[25] The *qichong* point: ST-30 who, i.e., *Qi* Thoroughfare; five thumb-widths below the umbilicus, two thumb-widths away from the ventro-medial line.

[26] The *biguan* point: ST-31 who, i.e., Thigh Joint; on the connecting line of the anterior superior iliac spine and the outer edge of the patella, level with the bottom line of the hip.

[27] The *futu* point: ST-32 who, i.e., Crouching Rabbit; on the connecting line of the anterior superior iliac spine and the outer edge of the patella, six thumb-widths above the outer edge of the patella.

[28] *Qi* reversal of the tibia: The bright-*yang* stomach channel descends along the front edge of the outer side of the tibia, so the disease is named in this way.

[29] The channel dominates diseases due to disorders of the blood: The stomach is the sea of water and grains, and it dominates the production of blood. If the stomach is ill, the blood will not be produced.

[30] Mania, warm malaria, sweating: Because the stomach *qi* is hot, and it steams water.

[31] The foot greater-*yin* spleen channel: Abbreviated as the SP channel.

[32] The nut-like bone: The process of the metatarsal bone behind the big toe with the appearance of a nut.

[33] Loose stool, conglomeration, diarrhea, obstruction of urine, jaundice, inability to lie: When the spleen is cold, it causes loose stool and diarrhea. When the spleen *qi* is stagnant, it causes conglomeration (tumors). When the ill spleen fails to control water, diarrhea, obstruction, jaundice, and inability to lie appear.

[34] The hand lesser-*yin* heart channel: Abbreviated as the HT channel.

[35] The heart system: In this context, the network-channels that connect with the heart and other organs.

[36] The eye system: In this context, the network-channels that connect with the eyes and brain.

[37] The hand greater-*yang* small-intestine channel: Abbreviated as the SI channel.

[38] The two bones: The ulna and humerus.

[39] The small-intestine channel dominates diseases due to disorders of the fluids: The small-intestine dominates separating and filtering clearness and turbidity. If the small-intestine is ill, water and grains will not be separated.

[40] The foot greater-*yang* bladder channel: Abbreviated as the BL channel.

[41] *Qi*-surging headache: Evil *qi* surges upward to cause headache.

[42] The channel dominates diseases due to disorders of the tendons: When the *yang qi* is soft, it nourishes the tendons. The *qi* of the greater-*yang* is the leading *qi* among all *yang qi*. If the *yang* of the greater-*yang* bladder channel is insufficient, all tendons will fail to be nourished.

[43] The foot lesser-*yin* kidney channel: Abbreviated as the KI channel.

[44] The *rangu* point: KI-2 who, i.e., Blazing Vally; in the depression under the lower edge of the first process of the foot navicular.

[45] The disease is called *qi* reversal of the bone: The kidneys dominate the bones.

[46] *Qi* ascent: i.e., cough, hiccup or eructation.

[47] Intestinal flux: Diarrhea with pus and blood.

[48] Moxibustion could enhance the patient's appetite, and rich flavors can promote the growth of

muscles. The patient should loosen his laces, wear the hair down, and walk leisurely holding a big cane and wearing heavy shoes: Rich foods can promote the muscles to grow. Loosening laces and wearing the hair down and walking leisurely with a big cane and heavy shoes mean reducing work and nourishing the *qi*. Only in reference to this channel has the author mentioned these methods, because the true *yin* exists in the kidneys, and the essence is the root of the original *qi*.

[49] The hand cold-*yin* pericardium channel: Abbreviated as the PC channel.

[50] Connects with the three warmers, in order: Connects with the upper-warmer, middle-warmer and lower-warmer from the upper part to the lower part, in that order.

[51] The channel dominates diseases due to disorders of the vessels: The heart dominates the vessels, and the pericardium is the external fence of the heart, so the pericardium contracts evils instead of the heart. Therefore, the pericardium dominates diseases due to disorders of the vessels.

[52] The hand lesser-*yang* triple-warmer channel: Abbreviated as the TW channel.

[53] The two fingers: The third finger and little finger.

[54] The two bones: The ulna and the radius.

[55] The *shangguan* point: GB-3 who, i.e., Upper Gate.

[56] The channel dominates diseases due to disorders of the *qi*: The triple-warmer dominates the *qi* transformation of the whole body. The famous medical book, *Nanjing* (The Medical Classic on Eighty-One Difficult Questions), says that "the triple-warmer is the way of water and grains, and the end and beginning of the *qi*," and regards that "the triple-warmer is another envoy of the original *qi*, and it presides over all *qi*."

[57] The foot lesser-*yang* gallbladder channel: abbreviated as the GB channel.

[58] His face is slightly dust-covered: The face feels murky, as though covered by dust.

[59] The disease is called *qi* reversal of *yang*: This refers to disease due to *qi* reversal of the foot lesser-*yang*.

[60] Diseases due to disorders of the bones: Because the bones and tendons are homologous.

[61] Sabre-shaped and connecting pear-shaped scrofula: The sabre-shaped scrofula usually appears at the armpits. The connecting pear-shaped scrofula usually appears at the sides of the neck.

[62] The foot cold-*yin* liver channel: Abbreviated as the LV channel.

[63] Male prominent hernia: A disease name. Cold evil attacks the liver channel and kidney channel. The blood becomes stagnated inside. The lower abdomen becomes spasmodic and painful. The pains draw the testicles. In another case, the lower abdomen has masses that wrap pus and blood inside.

[64] Fox hernia: Due to failure of the dredging of the liver *qi*. When the disease is in onset, a part of small-intestine falls into the scrotum. It can return to the abdomen if the patient lies flat or if it is pushed by hands; yet it falls again if the patient stands up. Because it moves up and down, appearing and then disappearing as a fox prowls, the disease is named "fox hernia."

3.1.3   Original article

"The twelve main channels run latently in the muscles. They are deep and invisible. What can be seen is usually where the foot greater-*yin* spleen channel passes the medial malleolus. It is not hidden there. The floating and usually-seen parts are all network-channels. The large network-channels of the hand bright-*yang* channel and hand lesser-*yang* channel among the network-channels of the six hand channels[1] start amid the five fingers, ascend, and merge at the elbow.

"After one takes wine, the defensive *qi* runs first in the skin and fills the network-channels first. The network-channels become prosperous first. Hence, the defensive *qi* has become exuberant; then the nutritive *qi* becomes full, and the channels become extremely prosperous. If a channel has a sudden variation, evils have dwelled in it and stayed at its root and tip. If the channel has no sudden variation, there may be a fever.[2] If the channel is not shown solid, the evils must have sunk, and the channel is found empty. Because disordered channels differ from normal ones, the doctor can tell which channel has got a variation."

Lei Gong asked: "How can we know the difference between the channels and network-channels?"

The Emperor answered: "The channels are ordinarily invisible. Their deficiencies and excesses are also detected at the wrist pulse. The visible parts are all network-channels."

Lei Gong said: "I do not understand why that is so."

The Emperor explained: "None of the network-channels can bridge the gaps of the big joints. They must go other ways[3] and merge in the skin; so their meeting places are revealed outside. When needling a network-channel, the doctor should acupuncture the blood knots of the network-channel. If the blood is excessive, though there is not a knot, the doctor should quickly treat the network-channel to discharge the evils and allow it to bleed, otherwise impediment will occur if the evils stay.

"In all observations of the network-channels, the blue color of the network-channels indicates cold and pain, and the red color indicates heat. When there is cold in the stomach, the network-channels of the fish-abdomen-style muscles of the palms are mostly blue.[4] When there is heat in the stomach, they are red. If the network-channels suddenly go black, they reveal a long-resident impediment disease. If the network-channels are red and black and blue, cold and heat co-exist. If there are short blue network-channels, the *qi* is scanty. Shallowly needling the network-channels is the ordinary method to treat the cold and heat. The doctor should treat once every other day, stop needling when the blood is completely drained there, and then adjust the deficiency or excess. The patient with small, short network-channels lacks the *qi*. He may experience suffocation when bled excessively. Serious suffocation may lead to faintness and inability to speak. The doctor should quickly make the patient sit if he feels faint."

Commentary

The article mainly discusses the difference between the channels and network-channels, and the diagnostic and needling methods of the network-channels. The distinction between the channels and network-channels was proved by the separate treatments of channels and network-channels presented by the medical master, Ye Tianshi who lived in the Jin-Yuan Period, roughly 1115-1368.

Dr. Ye regarded that "the channels dominate the *qi*, while the network-channels dominate the blood," and "a new disease is at the channels, while an old disease gets into the network-channels." Therefore, his therapeutic method for the disordered network-channels is basically "quickening blood circulation and transforming stasis."

The network-channels, while they are different from the channels, have indivisible links with the channels. Their physiological functioning is to supplement the shortages of the twelve main channels, and act as important hubs, in order to make the running of the *qi* and blood smooth, and to make the communications of all human organs more organic and coherent. So, an ancient medical master said: "The (visible) blood networks are the superficial network-channels and grandchild network-channels shown at the skin. If the blood and *qi* stay and accumulate somewhat, the mechanism of getting in and getting out will fail."

The discussed diagnostic and needling methods of the network-channels have directive roles in clinical practice. Among these, the observation of the fish-abdomen-style muscles of the palms can help to diagnose the cold and heat and impediment, and to detect the waxing or waning of the stomach *qi*.

The article suggests in the end that, when a doctor meets a patient with poor constitution and deficient *qi*, he does well not to insert needles rashly, or the *qi* of the patient may become more deficient after drainage, and the patient may faint. In this situation, the doctor must stop needling quickly and allow the patient to calm down while supported in a sitting position. (It may be better for the patient to lie flat.) No physician can afford to ignore this warning in clinical practice.

Annotation

[1] The large network-channels of the hand bright-*yang* channel and hand lesser-*yang* channel among the network-channels of the six hand channels: Here the doctor should take the largest hand network-channels to demonstrate the method of observing the network-channels. The network-channels of the hand bright-*yang* channel and hand lesser-*yang* channel are the largest among all network-channels of the six hand channels.

[2] If the channel has no sudden variation, there may be a fever: In this case, the channel has not had a sudden variation, showing that evils are still at the shallow parts. Thus, there may be a fever.

[3] They must go other ways: They must take paths that the channels do not go through.

[4] When there is cold in the stomach, the network-channels of the fish-abdomen-style muscles of the palms are mostly blue: The cold makes the *qi* and blood congeal and stagnate, so the network-channels there are mostly blue. Though the fish-abdomen-style muscles of the palms are where the hand greater-*yin* lung channel passes, the stomach *qi* reaches the hand greater-*yin* lung channel. So, the stomach *qi* can be detected here.

3.1.4 Original article

"The branched network-channel of the hand greater-*yin* lung channel diverges at the *lieque* point.[1] It starts from the seam of muscles above the wrist, runs directly into the palm alongside with the greater-*yin* lung channel, and spreads into the fish-abdomen-style muscles. Its repletion disorders are hot ulnar processes near the wrists and hot palms. Its vacuity disorders are yawning and urinary incontinence or frequent urination. Find it one and a half thumb-widths away from the wrist. Its diverged line runs to the hand bright-*yang* channel.

"The branched network-channel of the hand lesser-*yin* heart channel diverges at the *tongli* point[2] that is a thumb-width away from the wrist, ascends and moves along the heart channel to get into the heart, and connects with the tongue root and eye system. Its repletion disorder is propped diaphragm.[3] Its vacuity disorder is inability to speak. Find it a thumb-width above the palm. Its diverged line runs to the hand greater-*yang* channel.

"The branched network-channel of the hand cold-*yin* pericardium channel diverges at the *neiguan* point[4] that is two thumb-widths away from the wrist, gets out between the two tendons, moves upward with the pericardium channel, and connects with the pericardium and heart system. Its repletion disorder is painful heart. Its vacuity disorder is vexation. Find it between the two tendons.

"The branched network-channel of the hand greater-*yang* small-intestine channel diverges at the *zhizheng* point[5] that is five thumb-widths away from the wrist. Its diverged line rushes into the hand lesser-*yin* channel. Its branch ascends upward to the elbow, and connects with the *jianyu* point[6] of the shoulder. Its repletion disorders are flaccid joints and disabled elbows. Its vacuity disorder is warts with small ones looking like scabs on the fingers. Use this point.

"The branched network-channel of the hand bright-*yang* large-intestine channel diverges at the *pianli* point[7] that is three thumb-widths away from the wrist. Its diverged line gets into the hand greater-*yin* lung channel.

"Its branch ascends along the arm, mounts the *jianyu* point, ascends the corner of the lower jaw, and connects with the root of the teeth. Its continuous branch gets into the ear and merges with the ancestral channel.[8] Its repletion disorders are dental caries and deafness. Its vacuity disorders are cold teeth and numb and blockaded gums. Use this point.

"The branched network-channel of the hand lesser-*yang* triple-warmer channel diverges at the *waiguan* point[9] that is two thumb-widths away from the wrist, gets around the outer side of the arm, rushes into the chest, and merges with the pericardium. Its repletion disorder is spasmodic elbows. Its vacuity disorder is inability to flex the elbows. Use this point.

"The branched network-channel of the foot greater-*yang* bladder channel diverges at the *feiyang* point[10] that is seven thumb-widths away from the ankle. Its diverged line runs to the foot lesser-*yin* channel. Its repletion disorders are nasal congestion and painful head and back. Its vacuity disorder is nasal congestion and nosebleed. Use this point.

"The branched network-channel of the foot lesser-*yang* gallbladder channel diverges at the *guangming* point[11] that is five thumb-widths away from the ankle. Its diverged line runs to the foot cold-*yin* channel. The network-channel descends to connect with the instep. It repletion disorder is *qi* reversal. Its vacuity disorders are limp atrophy and inability to get up from a sitting position. Use this point.

"The branched network-channel of the foot bright-*yang* stomach channel diverges at the *fenglong* point[12] that is eight thumb-widths away from the ankle. Its diverged line runs to the foot greater-*yin* channel. Its branch moves along the outer edge of the tibia, ascends to connect with the head and neck, merges with the *qi* of all channels,[13] and descends to connect with the throat. If the *qi* is reverse, numb throat and sudden inability to speak will occur. Its repletion disorders are mania and madness. Its vacuity disorders are inability to flex the legs and withered shanks. Use this point.

"The branched network-channel of the foot greater-*yin* spleen channel diverges at the *gongsun* point[14] that is a thumb-width away from the end of the great toe. Its diverged line runs to the foot bright-*yang* channel. Its branch gets in to connect with the intestines and stomach. If the disordered *qi* ascends adversely, sudden turmoil[15] will occur. Its repletion disorder is cutting pain in the intestines. Its vacuity disorder is drum distention. Use this point.

"The branched network-channel of the foot lesser-*yin* kidney channel diverges at the *dazhong* point.[16] It gets around the heel after the medial malleolus. Its diverged line runs to the foot greater-*yang* channel. Its branch ascends with the kidney channel to the pericardium, and descends outward to penetrate the loin and spine. If its *qi* is reverse, vexation and depression will occur. Its repletion disorder is urinary blockade. Its vacuity disorder is painful loins. Use this point.

"The branched network-channel of the foot cold-*yin* liver channel diverges at the *ligou* point[17] that is five thumb-widths away from the medial malleolus. Its diverged line runs to the foot lesser-*yang* channel. Its branch ascends to the testicle with the liver channel, and ends at the penis. If its *qi* is reverse, swollen testicles and sudden hernia will occur. Its repletion disorder is erect and long penis. Its vacuity disorder is sudden genital itching. Use this point.

"The branched network-channel of the controlling channel diverges at the *jiuwei* point[18] that is under the xiphoid, and spreads in the abdomen. Its repletion disorder is pain of the ventral skin. Its vacuity disorder is itching of the same area. Use this point.

"The branched network-channel of the governing channel diverges at the *changqiang* point,[19] clamps the muscles beside the spine, ascends the neck, spreads at the head top, descends to the area between the scapulas, diverges into two lines to run to the foot greater-*yang* channel, and gets in to penetrate through the spine. Its repletion disorder is stiff spine. Its vacuity disorders are heavy head and shaking highly of the head because the network-channel that clamps the spine is disordered. Use this point.

"The big network-channel of the spleen diverges at the *dabao* point[20] that is three thumb-widths below the *yuanye* point,[21] and spreads at the chest and rib-side. Its repletion disorder is generalized pain. Its vacuity disorder is flaccidity of all the body's joints. The big network-channel of the spleen seems to wrap blood of all network-channels. Use the big network-channel of the spleen itself.

"All these fifteen branched network-channels, when replete, must be visible; when vacuous, must be deep and invisible. Doctors should seek up and down carefully, because the channels of human bodies vary greatly, and the precise location of the network-channels may vary as well."

Commentary

This article discusses the names, locations, running routes, and replete and vacuous signs of the fifteen branched network-channels, an important subject in the syndrome identification of channels and network-channels. The fifteen branched network-channels that branch from the fourteen channels are different from other common network-channels. They possess special functions in physiology. They are the hubs of the *yin* channels and *yang* channels of the interior and exterior. The article suggests that the channels of human bodies vary greatly. So we must adhere to the principle of "taking different measures to different individuals" in analyzing physiology and pathology, and thinking about syndrome identification and treatment.

There are points on each of the fifteen branched network-channels that have therapeutic roles in diagnosing deficiency syndrome or excess syndrome of that channel, because they possess the ability to adjust the channel *qi* of *yin* and *yang*.

Annotation

[1] The *lieque* point: LU-7 who, i.e., Broken Sequence. It pertains to the hand greater-*yin* lung channel, one and a half thumb-widths away from the transverse crease of the wrist.

[2] The *tongli* point: HT-5 who, i.e., Connecting Inside.

[3] Propped diaphragm: The term "propped diaphragm" is a subjective symptom. The patient feels a sensation of propping up and discomfort in the chest and diaphragm.

[4] The *neiguan* point: PC-6 who, i.e., Inner Pass.

[5] The *zhizheng* point: SI-7 who, i.e., Branch to the Correct.

[6] The *jianyu* point: LI-15 who, i.e., Shoulder Bone. It pertains to the hand bright-*yang* large-intestine channel, in the anterior depression of the shoulder when the arm is lifted up horizontally.

[7] The *pianli* point: LI-6 who, i.e., Veering Passage-way.

[8] The ancestral channel: Refers to the big channel made by the convergence of many channels; the hand greater-*yang*, hand lesser-*yang*, foot lesser-*yang* and foot bright-*yang*, all converge in the ear.

[9] The *waiguan* point: TW-5, i.e., Outer Pass.

[10] The *feiyang* point: BL-58 who, i.e., Taking Flight.

[11] The *guangming* point: GB-37 who, i.e., Bright Light.

[12] The *fenglong* point: ST-40 who, i.e., Bountiful Bulge.

[13] Merges with the *qi* of all channels: The *qi* and blood of the fifteen branched network-channels stem from water and grains in the stomach. So we say that the branched network-channel of the foot bright-*yang* stomach channel merges with the *qi* of all channels.

[14] The *gongsun* point: SP-4 who, i.e., Yellow Emperor.

[15] Sudden turmoil: It is used as a disease name; its symptoms are sudden effusive vomiting and diarrhea.

[16] The *dazhong* point: KI-4 who, i.e., Large Goblet.

[17] The *ligou* point: LV-5, i.e., Woodworm Canal.

[18] The *jiuwei* point: Also known as CV-15 who, Turtledove Tail.

[19] The *changqiang* point: Also known as GV-1 who, i.e., Long Strong. It pertains to the governing channel, at the back edge of the perineum.

[20] The *dabao* point: SP-21 who, Great Embracement.

[21] The *yuanye* point: GB-22 who, i.e., Armpit Abyss. It pertains to the foot lesser-*yang* gallbladder channel, three thumb-widths below the armpit, on the median line of the flank, at the fifth intercostal space.

3.2   Sixteenth Article

Nutritive Qi · The Divine Pivot

Original article

The Emperor said:

To the running of the nutritive *qi*, taking grains is precious.[1] Grains enter the stomach, the essential *qi* is transmitted to the lungs. The *qi* flows and spills inside, and spreads outside. The essential *qi* runs in the channels, and acts endlessly. The circulation repeats perpetually. It is called rule of the heaven and earth.

So, the *qi* starts to run from the hand greater-*yin* lung channel, rushes into the hand bright-*yang* large-intestine channel, ascends to rush into the foot bright-*yang* stomach channel, descends to the instep, rushes into the great toe to merge with the foot greater-*yin* spleen channel, and runs upward to reach the spleen. The *qi* rushes into the heart from the spleen, moves along the hand lesser-*yin* heart channel to get out of the armpit and descend the arm, rushes into the little finger to merge with the hand greater-*yang* small-intestine channel, ascends to mount the shoulder and get out of the region below the eye socket, rushes into the inner canthus, mounts the vertex, and descends the neck to merge with the foot greater-*yang* bladder channel.

Continuing, it moves along the spine to descend the buttock, runs downward to rush to the end of the little toe, moves through the center of the sole to rush into the foot lesser-*yin* kidney channel, runs upward into the kidney, rushes into the heart from the kidney, and spreads outward in the chest.

The *qi* then moves along the hand cold-*yin* pericardium channel to get out of the armpit and descend the arm, gets out between the two tendons, gets into the palm, gets out of the end of the middle finger, returns to rush into the end of the third finger, merges with the hand lesser-*yang* triple-warmer channel, ascends to rush into the chest, spreads at the triple-warmer, rushes into the gallbladder from the triple-warmer, gets out of the rib-side, and rushes into the foot lesser-*yang* gallbladder channel.

Still continuing, it runs downward to the instep, rushes into the great toe from the instep again, merges with the foot cold-*yin* liver channel, ascends to the liver, rushes upward into the lung from the liver, ascends along the throat, gets into the palate, and ends at the nostrils.

Its branch ascends the forehead, moves along the vertex, descends the median line of the nape, moves along the spine, and gets into the sacrum. This is the passage of the governing channel.

Another branch connects with the genitals, ascends to pass the pubes, gets into the umbilicus, ascends along the inside of the abdomen, gets into the supraclavicular fossa, rushes downward into the lung, and gets out of the hand greater-*yin* lung channel again. This is the running route of the nutritive *qi*. The normal routine is this.

Commentary

This section describes the running route and regularity of the nutritive *qi* in the body. We can see that the running route of the nutritive *qi* is identical to the running sequence of the twelve main channels, i. e., from the lung channel to the large-intestine channel, stomach channel, spleen channel, heart channel, small-intestine channel, bladder channel, kidney channel, pericardium channel, triple-warmer channel, gallbladder channel, and liver channel, in that order. The only difference is that the running route of the nutritive *qi* diverges at the liver, ascends to the forehead and vertex, descends the neck to get into the governing channel, gets around the genitals to cross the controlling channel, and rushes into the lung from the controlling channel. Then a new circulation begins.

The article mentions that taking grains is precious to the nutritive *qi*, because the nutritive *qi* comes from the essence of grains produced by the stomach and spleen, enabling the nutritive *qi* to circulate and run perpetually. This proposition presents a reference for curing insufficiency of the nutritive blood by focusing on the spleen and stomach in clinical practice.

Annotation

[1] To the running of the nutritive *qi*, taking grains is precious: If grains cannot be taken, the lack of sustenance will enfeeble the nutritive *qi*.

3.3   Seventy-eighth Article

Discussion of Nine Needles · The Divine Pivot (excerpt)

Original article

The bright-*yang* channels have copious *qi* and copious blood. The greater-*yang* channels have copious blood and scant *qi*. The lesser-*yang* channels have copious *qi* and scant blood. The greater-*yin* channels have copious blood and scant *qi*. The cold-*yin* channels have copious blood and scant *qi*. The lesser-*yin* channels have copious *qi* and scant blood.

So we say that needling the bright-*yang* channels to drain their blood and *qi* is proper. Needling the greater-*yang* channels to drain their blood is proper, yet the drainage of *qi* is improper. Needling the lesser-*yang* channels to drain their *qi* is proper, yet the drainage of the blood is improper. Needle the greater-*yin* channels to drain the blood, not the *qi*. Needle the cold-*yin* channels to drain the blood, not the *qi*. Needle the lesser-*yin* channels to drain the *qi*, not the blood.

The foot bright-*yang* stomach channel and foot greater-*yin* spleen channel are exterior-interior. The foot lesser-*yang* gallbladder channel and foot cold-*yin* liver channel are exterior-interior. The foot greater-*yang* bladder channel and foot lesser-*yin* kidney channel are exterior-interior. These are the correspondences of *yin* and *yang* of the foot channels. The hand bright-*yang* large-intestine channel and hand greater-*yin* lung channel are exterior-interior. The hand lesser-*yang* triple-warmer channel and hand cold-*yin* pericardium channel are exterior-interior. The hand greater-*yang* small-intestine channel and hand lesser-*yin* heart channel are exterior-interior. These are the correspondences of *yin* and *yang* of the hand channels.

Commentary

This section discusses the amounts of the *qi* and blood in the twelve main channels, and the cooperative relationships of exterior and interior between the *yin* channels and *yang* channels. These are significant to clinical syndrome identifications, especially to needling treatment. In acupuncture practice, physicians should take careful note of the amounts of the *qi* and blood in the channels when they needle to supplement the deficiency or to drain the excess. The copious one may be drained, yet the scant one should not be drained. Every couple of cooperative *yin* and *yang* channels can affect each other in pathological changes. So, when a *yang* channel is disordered, the points of its corresponding *yin* channel can be needled cooperatively, and vice versa. The effect can be remarkably improved.

In this section, the copious or scant amounts of the *qi* and blood in the twelve main channels are slightly different from what is described in other sections of *The Medical Classic of the Yellow Emperor*.

3.4   Fifty-first Article

Back Transport Points · The Divine Pivot (*excerpt*)

Original article

The Emperor asked Uncle Qi: "Please tell me the transport points of the five *zang*-organs[1] that are at the back."

Uncle Qi answered: "The chest transport point[2] is under the spinal process of the first thoracic vertebra. The lung transport point is under the spinal process of the third thoracic vertebra. The heart transport point is under the spinal process of the fifth thoracic vertebra. The diaphragm transport point is under that of the seventh thoracic vertebra. The liver transport point is under that of the ninth thoracic vertebra. The spleen transport point is under that of the eleventh thoracic vertebra. The kidney transport point is under that of the second lumbar vertebra. All these points[3] are one and a half thumb-widths away from the spine. To prove this, press that point — if the pain inside is relieved correspondingly, that is the transport point.[4]"

Commentary

This section discusses the transport points of the five *zang*-organs located on the foot bright-*yang* stomach channel on the back. The *qi* of a *zang*-organ converges at a corresponding transport point. So, when a *zang*-organ is ill, the illness will be shown there clearly. However, since the channels of human bodies vary greatly, different patients will have somewhat different locations of the *zang-fu* organs and different-sized organs, so the transport points may also be different. We should seek for them at their appropriate places. Press that aching point, if the pain inside is relieved correspondingly, or if the patient feels distention or aching, the transport point is then determined. This method of point selection is called "taking the painful place as the point" and "taking the pleasant place as the point."

Using this theory, some physicians selected a number of typical cases that had been definitely diagnosed, and compared the concerned channels and points that have therapeutic roles to those diseases. They deliberately sought for these points and their regularities. They found a few intrinsic relationships between some commonly encountered diseases and the reactions of tenderness at certain points. So they further regarded the reactions of tenderness at these points as a diagnostic indication. Inserting needles at these points with apparent tenderness can bring about strong needling reaction and good effect.

Annotation

[1] The transport points of the five *zang*-organs: Every *zang*-organ or *fu*-organ can transport its channel *qi* to a point on the stomach channel. This back point can reflect the condition of its concerned *zang*-organ or *fu*-organ.

[2] The chest transport point: i.e., the *dazhu* point (BL-11 who, or Great Shuttle).

[3] All these points: Located on the foot bright-*yang* stomach channel.

[4] To prove this, press that point — if the pain inside is relieved correspondingly, that is the transport point: Another proof is to press that point, and if the patient feels distention and aching, that is the transport point.

3.5   Sixtieth Article

Discussion of Holes in Bones · The Plain Questions (*excerpt*)

Original article

The controlling channel starts under the *zhongji* point,[1] ascends the pubic region, moves along the ventro-medial line, ascends the *guanyuan* point,[2] reaches the throat, ascends the cheek, and moves along the face to get into the eye. The penetrating channel passes the *qichong* point, runs together with the foot lesser-*yin* kidney channel, ascends clamping the navel, and spreads inside the chest. When the controlling channel has been disordered, the male patient suffers from all types of hernias; and the female patient suffers from abnormal leucorrhoea and conglomeration and gathering. When the penetrating channel has been disordered, the patient suffers from adverse *qi* and urgent abdomen.[3]

When the governing channel has been disordered, the spine becomes stiff and bends backward. The governing channel starts from the anterior center of the pubic bone below the lower abdomen. In females, the governing channel gets in to connect with the urinary gate, i.e., the mouth of the urethra. Its network-channel moves along the genitals, merges at the perineum, and gets around to the back of the perineum. Its branch gets around the hip, and reaches the foot lesser-*yin* channel to merge with the middle network-channel of the foot greater-*yang* bladder channel. The foot lesser-*yin* channel ascends the back edge of the inner face of the thigh. Its branch penetrates the spine and connects with the kidney.

Its continuous branch starts from the inner canthus with the foot greater-*yang* bladder channel, ascends the forehead, crosses at the vertex, gets in to connect with the brain, returns out, descends the neck, moves along the inner side of the scapula, clamps the spine, reaches the loin, gets in to move through the muscles beside the spine, and links up with the kidney. In males, the governing channel descends along the penis to reach the perineum. The remainder of the route is identical to that in females. Another branch of the governing channel ascends directly from the lower abdomen, penetrates the center of the navel, ascends to penetrate the heart, gets into the throat, ascends the cheek, gets around the lips, and ascends to link up with the centers under the two eyes.

When the governing channel has been disordered, the *qi* surges upward to the heart to induce pain, and the patient cannot urinate or defecate. The disease is called surging hernia. The female patient may suffer from sterility, obstructed urine, hemorrhoid, bedwetting, and a dry throat.

Commentary

This section describes the running routes of the controlling channel, penetrating channel and governing channel, and their commonly encountered diseases. From the angle of the syndrome identification of peculiar channels, the article provides references to diagnosing chronic or difficult diseases in clinical internal medicine and gynecology, especially to treating diseases of pregnancy, delivery and menstruation.

The article mentions that the three peculiar channels, i.e., the controlling channel, penetrating channel and governing channel, all start from the lower abdomen, get out of the perineum, ascend the ventro-median line, or the two sides of the abdomen, or the median line of the back. They are of the same source, with three different branches. So regarding physiology and pathology, they have intrinsic relationships.

In clinical practice, when we use the theory of these three peculiar channels to direct the practice, the concerned organs should be considered in combination. The real cause of occurrence can then be determined. Furthermore, we should pay acute attention to the links between these three channels and other main channels. Take the penetrating channel as an example: Because the penetrating channel is widespread, it is also called "the sea of the twelve main channels." In these twelve main channels, the penetrating channel is closer to the foot lesser-*yin* kidney channel and foot bright-*yang* stomach channel, because the penetrating channel merges with the foot lesser-*yin* kidney channel and links up with the foot bright-*yang* stomach channel.

Thus, physicians can achieve a better comprehension of the physiology of the penetrating channel and concerned pathomechanism. It is also profitable for physicians to understand the design of therapeutic methods in gynecological diseases, and the therapeutic methods and prescriptions of their predecessors.

As to the running route of the penetrating channel, the descriptions in a number of articles of *The Medical Classic of the Yellow Emperor* are not at all identical, so physicians need to consider them in combination.

Annotation

[1] The *zhongji* point: Also known as CV-3 who, i.e., Central Pole; four thumb-widths below

the umbilicus on the perpendicular.

[2] The *guanyuan* point: Also known as CV-4 who, i.e., Pass Head; three thumb-widths below the umbilicus perpendicularly.

[3] Urgent abdomen: Painful abdomen.

3.6   **Thirty-eighth Article**
Unfavorableness, Favorableness, Thickness, and Thinness ·
The Divine Pivot (excerpt)

Original article

The Emperor asked: "Why does only the foot lesser-*yin* kidney channel run downward?[1]"

Uncle Qi answered: "No, it does not run downward. The penetrating channel is the sea of the five *zang*-organs and six *fu*-organs. The five *zang*-organs and six *fu*-organs are all bestowed with *qi* from that channel. Its upper branch gets out of the palate, permeates all *yang* channels, and irrigates them with essential *qi*. Its lower branch rushes into the large network-channel of the foot lesser-*yin* kidney channel, gets out of the *qichong* point, moves along the inner face of the thigh, gets into the hollow of the knee, runs latently inside the tibia, descends to reach where the medial malleolus connect with the metatarsal bones, and diverges into two lines.

"The lower line merges with the foot lesser-*yin* kidney channel, and permeates the three *yin* channels. The front line runs latently to get out of the instep, descends along the instep to get into the great toe, permeates all the network-channels, and warms the muscles."

Commentary

This section particularly describes the running route of the penetrating channel and its physiological functions, and presents that the penetrating channel is the sea of the five *zang*-organs and six *fu*-organs. This proposition had a far-reaching influence in later periods of time. The penetrating channel generally commands the *qi* and blood of all channels. The channel reaches the head upward and the feet downward. It can regulate the *qi* and blood of the twelve main channels, irrigate all *yang* channels at the upper part of the body, and permeate all *yin* channels at the lower part of the body. Therefore, the penetrating channel is also called "the sea of the twelve channels" and "the sea of blood."

Annotation

[1] Why does only the foot lesser-*yin* kidney channel run downward: Here, the foot lesser-*yin* kidney channel should be the penetrating channel. All foot *yin* channels run from the feet to the abdomen. The fact that the penetrating channel rushes into the network-channel of the foot lesser-*yin* kidney channel and runs along with it makes it difficult to distinguish between them.

3.7　Seventeenth Article

Measurements of the Channels · The Divine Pivot (excerpt)

Original article

The Emperor asked: "Where do the springing channels[1] start and end? Which channel *qi* nourishes them?[2]"

Uncle Qi answered: "The *yin*-springing channel diverging from the foot lesser-*yin* kidney channel starts from the *zhaohai* point[3] after the *rangu* point.[4] It ascends above the medial malleolus, ascends directly, moves along the inner face of the thigh to get into the genitals, ascends along the inner side of the breast to get into the supraclavicular fossa, ascends to get out before the *renying* point, gets into the region below the eye, and connects with the inner canthus to merge with the foot greater-*yang* bladder channel.

"The *yang*-springing channel ascends. The *qi* of the *yin*-springing channel and *yang*-springing channel merges at the inner canthus, gets around the eye and nourishes it. If that *qi* is not flourishing, the eyes cannot close."

The Emperor asked: "Why does the *qi* of the *yin*-springing channel run only in the five *zang*-organs, and not nourish the six *fu*-organs?"

Uncle Qi answered: "The *qi* cannot stand still. It runs like the flowing of water and the endless movement of the sun and moon. Therefore, the *yin*-springing channel nourishes the *zang*-organs, and the *yang* – springing channel nourishes the *fu*-organs in an endless lope. The exact schedule remains unknown, and a new circulation begins when the old one terminates. The overflowing *qi* of the springing channels irrigates the *zang-fu* organs inside and moistens the muscular striae outside."

The Emperor asked: "The springing channels include the *yin* and *yang*. Whose length is calculated by the channels?[5]"

Uncle Qi answered: "The *yang*-springing channel is assigned to men. The *yin*-springing channel is assigned to women. The assigned one is their channel, and the other is their network-channel."

Commentary

This section talks about the springing channels and their functions. It points out that men put the *yang*-springing as their channel, whereas women put the *yin*-springing as their channel. The *yin*-springing channel diverging from the foot lesser-*yin* kidney channel starts from the *zhaohai* point under the medial malleolus, and ascends along the medial malleolus. The *yang*-springing channel diverging from the foot greater-*yang* bladder channel starts from the *shenmai* point (BL-62 who, i.e., Extending Vessel), and ascends along the lateral malleolus. The two channels all reach the inner canthus, and are pertinent to the opening and closing of the eyes. The getting in and out and the crossing of the two channels have the functions of irrigating the *zang-fu* organs inside and moistening the muscular striae outside.

Annotation

[1] The springing channels: Including the *yin*-springing channel and *yang*-springing channel.

[2] Which channel *qi* nourishes them: It means that whichever channel *qi* the springing channels depend on to run endlessly.

[3] The *zhaohai* point: KI-6 who, i.e., Shining Sea; exactly one thumb-width below the tip of the medial malleolus.

[4] The *rangu* point: KI-2 who, i.e., Blazing Vally.

[5] The springing channels include the *yin* and *yang*. Whose length is calculated by the channels: Men put the *yang*-springing as their channel, and the *yin*-springing as their network-channel. Women put the *yin*-springing as their channel, and the *yang*-springing as their network-channel. Only the length of a channel can be calculated inside the total length of all channels.

3.8   Twenty-first Article

Diseases with Chills and Fevers·
The Divine Pivot (*excerpt*)

Original article

The *yin*-springing channel and *yang*-springing channel crisscross. The *yang* gets into the *yin*, and the *yin* gets out of the *yang*. They cross at the inner canthus. When the *yang qi* is exuberant, a man opens the eyes. When the *yin qi* is exuberant, a man closes the eyes.

Commentary

This section manifests that the *yin*-springing channel and *yang*-springing cross at the inner canthus. The waxing or waning of these two channels is closely relevant to sleep. This condition provides a means of curing insomnia by the method of fostering *yin* and subduing *yang*.

Chapter Four
Theory of Pathogens and Pathomechanisms

The theory of pathogens encompasses research into all disease-causing factors, and their properties, assortments, and characteristics to induce diseases. This theory as described in *The Medical Classic of the Yellow Emperpor* is based upon the integral idea that man and nature are mutually interrelated. The theory's foundations are the theory of *yin-yang*, the theory of the five elements, the theory of *zang*-organs and manifestations, and the theory of channels and network-channels. It states that the causes of disease include the effect of exogenous evil; emotional disorder; intemperate diet; imbalanced daily life; physical, mental or sexual exhaustion; injury by fall, fracture, contusion or strain; and other such factors. Among these influences, the external factors invading the body pertain to the *yang*; the internal factors occurring inside pertain to the *yin*. Because there is wide variation in both the causes of disease and their manifestations, in clinical practice doctors need to synthesize all symptoms when determining a disease's ultimate cause. This approach is what is referred to as "ascertaining the symptoms to seek the cause."

The pathomechanism is the mechanism of occurrence, development, and change of a disease. The theory of pathomechanisms deals with the occurrence of disease, pathological change, transmission, etc. Pathomechanism comprises two parts. One is the general mechanism of all kinds of diseases, such as the conditions of occurrence, the unbalanced *yin* and *yang*, the changes of vacuity and repletion, the pathomechanisms of the *zang-fu* organs and channels, the rules of disease transmission, etc. The other is the concrete mechanism of every disease and symptom.

The theory of pathomechanisms as discussed in *The Medical Classic of the Yellow Emperor* places special emphasis on the roles of the patient's inner factors. It states that of the two sides of the right *qi* and evils, the right *qi* decides not only whether a disease will occur, but also its degree of seriousness, property of vacuity or repletion, and change; as well as whether a patient will recover. When analyzing the pathomechanism of a disease, doctors need to keep in mind two key ideas. One is that the human body is an integral entity, of which the *zang-fu* organs form the center. The other is that human physiological processes must constantly adapt to the natural circumstances in order to maintain balanced health. Therefore, while underscoring the important position of the five *zang*-organs and six *fu*-organs during the course of a disease, a doctor should not neglect the close relationship between the natural factors (such as the seasonal and climatic variations) and the course of the disease.

4.1   Third Article

Discussion of Vital-Qi Corresponding to the Heaven · The Plain Questions

4.1.1   Original article

The Emperor said:

From ancient times, people who knew the heavenly law realized that the basis of life is rooted in the *yin* and *yang*. Between the heaven and earth and in the six orientations,[1] the nine orifices, five *zang*-organs and twelve joints[2] all correspond to the *qi* of the *yin* and *yang* of nature, which yields the five elements and the three *qi*.[3] If the numbers infringe these (five or three), the evils will impair people. The *yin* and *yang* are the basis of life.

If the heavenly *qi* is clear, one's mental state will be sound. Obedience to it makes the *yang qi* secure. Though evils exist, they cannot poison men. These are actions responding to the orders of time. Therefore, sages concentrate their minds, acclimatize themselves to the heavenly *qi*, and integrate the *qi* of *yin* and *yang* of nature with their own. If one violates this principle, the nine orifices will be obstructed inside, the muscles will be congested outside, and the defensive *qi* will dissipate. This is called self-injury, for the *yang qi* has been consumed.

Commentary

This article is the guidelines for the following questions:

(1) What is the source of life? In medicine, the conflict between materialism and idealism has its root in the conflict of matter and spirit. This article shows explicitly and incontrovertibly that the basis of life is rooted in the *yin* and *yang*. Because the materialistic interpretation could be confirmed in the real world, the foundation and development of the theoretical system of TCM were greatly refined.

(2) Was the world created by a Supreme Being? No. The *qi* of the *yin* and *yang* of nature produced the five elements, and the *qi* of the three *yin* and three *yang*. That is to say, the *qi* of *yin* and *yang* of the cosmos made the world. This viewpoint dealt a heavy blow at the prevailing superstitious notions of a Creator.

Annotation

[1] The six orientations: i.e., the upward, downward, east, west, south, and north direc-

tions.

    [2] Twelve joints: The bilateral joints of the wrists, elbows, shoulders, ankles, knees, and hips.

    [3] The three *qi*: i.e., the *qi* of the three *yang* and three *yin*.

4.1.2 Original article

The *yang qi* is just like the sun in the sky. If the *yang qi* fails to run normally, one's life-span will be shortened and he will not be healthy. Therefore, the motions of the celestial bodies are normal due to the sunlight. By the same mechanism, the *yang qi* of a man runs upward, acting as a defensive force.

When one is attacked by cold, the defensive *qi* no longer moves flexibly as a pivot. The regular life becomes abnormal and the *yang qi* is depleted. When one is assailed by summer heat, perspiration occurs. The patient either has rough gasp when being vexed, or becomes delirious when being quiet.[1] The body is as hot as burning coal, and the *yang qi* evaporates along with perspiration. Hit by dampness, he feels his head wrapped. The dampness and heat cannot be dispelled. The large sinews shrink and turn shorter. The small sinews slacken and turn longer. The former condition induces cramp, and the next brings about atrophy. When he is assailed by wind, swelling ensues. The four evils assault him in alternation, eventually exhausting the *yang qi*.

Physical overstrain can make the *yang qi* overwhelming outside, and exhaust the *yin* essence inside. If this happens frequently till the summer comes, fried-coma[2] is caused. The eyes become blind and cannot see. The ears become deaf and cannot listen. Fried-coma seems like a collapsing dam, an overflowing deluge, and gurgling rapids that cannot be stopped. Rage can obstruct the *qi* of the body. The blood stagnates in the head, inducing oppressed-coma. The sinews are injured, and the limbs become flaccid and seemingly disabled. Perspiration happens over half of the body, and hemiplegia occurs. If the sweat encounters dampness, small furuncles and prickly heats will appear. The harm caused by greasy and fine foods[3] is enough to induce big malignant boils. It is as easy as holding a hollow vessel to receive things. If sweat is exposed to wind when one is working, the cold will settle. Small acnes, even small furuncles due to stagnation, will arise.

The *yang qi* nourishes the spirit to make it vigorous, and nourishes the sinews to make them lithe. When the defensive *qi* fails to open or close the skin's pores, cold intrudes and hunchback may occur. If the evil further sinks into the channels, fistulas will appear. The evil lingers in the muscular striae, and trespasses through the channels to oppress the five *zang*-organs. After transmission, susceptibility to fear and even fright may occur.[4] If the nutritive *qi* is disordered and enters the muscular striae adversely, carbuncles will ensue. The white perspiration[5] does not end, and the body form is gaunt. The *yang qi* is dissipated by heat, and the acupuncture points are closed. Then wind malaria[6] ensues.

Therefore, the wind is the beginning of the hundred diseases. If the *yang qi* is clear and serene, the muscular striae will be compact to repel. Even if there are great winds and pernicious evils, the body would not be poisoned. That is because he acclimatizes himself to the changes of seasons. So, if one is ill protractedly, the disease will worsen, and the *qi* of the upper part and lower part will not communicate. Even a proficient doctor can do nothing to resolve this condition. Thus, excessive amassment of the *yang qi* will kill a person. The measure of draining should be employed to dredge the amassment if the *yang qi* is blockaded, or the patient will not receive a timely, right treatment, and the inept practitioner will bungle the cure.

The *yang qi* dominates the outside in daytime. It engenders at dawn, and blooms at midday. When the *yang qi* has weakened at dusk, the sweat pores are closed. So, men should astringe the *yang qi* to repel evils after dusk.[7] Do not harass the sinews and bones, nor expose to dew or fog. If one infringes these rules of three times, the body form will become weary and weak.

Commentary

This article focuses upon the various symptoms and signs resulting from abnormalities of the *yang qi*, and their mechanisms. The *yang qi* of the body can be likened to the sun, showing the importance of the *yang qi*. Keeping copious *yang qi* is crucial to disease prevention and health maintenance. These ideas provided a theoretical reference for the medical school that attached importance to the *yang qi*. The medical master, Zhang Jiebin, postulated that "the great treasure of the sky is the sole sun, and the great treasure of a man is the sole genuine *yang*."

The two syndromes, fried-coma and oppressed-coma mentioned in the article, can be seen in clinical practice. Fried-coma is due to overstrain, which induces over-flourishing *yang* to destroy the *yin*. So, its pathomechanisms are failure of water to control fire, *yin* deficiency and flaring fire. Oppressed-coma is due to rage, which forces the *qi* and blood to rush recklessly upward. Thus, the former case is a vacuity syndrome, and the latter is a repletion syndrome.

The article elucidates the relationship between the *yang qi* of the body and the changes of the *yin* and *yang* of nature. It not only underscores the view that the *yang qi* corresponds to nature, but also points out that men should adapt to fluctuations in the *yin* and *yang* of nature so as to preserve health.

Annotation

[1] The patient either has rough gasp when being vexed, or becomes delirious when being quiet: The pathogenic heat evil from the aspect of the *qi* attacks the heart and vessels, so vexation occurs. The lungs are the cover of the heart. So the patient has rough gasp when being vexed. This condition is attributed to *yang* excess. When the heat evil subsequently injures the *yin*, delirium while quiet occurs. Quiet refers here to coma and somnolence. This condition is attributed to *yin* deficiency.

[2] Fried-coma: The *yang qi* prevails while the *yin* essence is exhausted, so deficient fire will be overwhelming. It seems as if the patient is fried by deficient heat evil, and coma occurs.

[3] The harm caused by greasy and fine foods: Taking too much fat meat and fine grains is apt to induce internal heat.

[4] After transmission, susceptibility to fear and even fright may occur: The *zang*-organs govern the storage of the spirit. They are damaged by evils, so the spirit is made uneasy. This suggests that the *yang qi* is harmed and fails to nourish the spirit.

[5] The white perspiration: i.e., spontaneous perspiration not due to heat.

[6] Wind malaria: Malaria due to wind evil.

[7] So, men should astringe the *yang qi* to repel evils after dusk: Reduce movement to store the *yang qi* so as to resist evils.

4.1.3　Original article

Uncle Qi said:

The *yin* stores the essence and rises frequently in response to the *yang* .[1] The *yang* defends and consolidates the outside for the *yin* .[2] If the *yin* cannot match the *yang* ,[3] the *qi* and blood will flow swiftly. When *yang* evils get into the *yang* aspect of the body, one will become mad.[4] If the *yang* cannot match the *yin*, the *qi* of the five *zang*-organs will not be in harmony and the nine orifices will become obstructed. Sages coordinate the *yin* and *yang* so that the sinews and channels are harmonious, the bones and marrow are solid, and the *qi* and blood are normal. In this way, the inside and outside will be harmonious, and evils will not poison people; the ears and eyes will be bright, and the *qi* will flow normally.

When wind evil intrudes upon the body, the *qi* becomes disordered, and the *yin* essence becomes dissipated.[5] As a result, the evil impairs the liver. During this time, if one overeats, the sinews and vessels will become flaccid. Intestinal flux[6] and hemorrhoid will ensue. If the patient consumes excess fluids, the *qi* will become disordered. If the patient indulges in sexual activity, the kidney *qi* will be damaged and the spine will be spoiled.

Generally, the crux of the *yin* and *yang* is that the *yang qi* is compact outside and the *yin qi* can then protect the inside firmly. If both lose the harmony, it is as if there is spring without autumn, and there is winter without summer. So, to harmonize the *yin* and *yang* is the policy of sages. If the *yang qi* is over-flourishing and fails to consolidate, the *yin qi* will be exhausted; if the *yin* and *yang* are in a harmonious balance, both essence and spirit will be normal; if the *yin* is severed from the *yang*, the essential *qi* will vanish.

If one is exposed to wind, chill and fever result. Hence, if one is spoiled by wind in the spring and the evil lingers, severe diarrhea will occur in the summer; if one is spoiled by summer heat in the summer, malaria will appear in the autumn; impaired by dampness in the autumn, the *qi* will rebel upward and produce cough, and atrophy diseases will ensue in the winter; impaired by cold in the winter, pyretic diseases will be bound to manifest in the spring. The evils of the four seasons harm the five *zang*-organs in alternation.

Commentary

This article develops further the relationship of mutual promotion and utilization between the *yang qi* and *yin* essence, and states that the *yin* is the basis of the *yang*, and the *yang* acts for the *yin*. This section enumerates the symptoms due to tendentious prosperity or decline, which is caused by disruption of this relationship, and describes how the harmonious *yin* and *yang* are the fundamental precondition that normalizes the functioning of the human body. The *yang qi* plays a leading role in the coordination of the *yin* and *yang*.

The last segment describes the concept of latent evil, offering a theoretical reference to the theory of latent evil found in later eras. It states that if the *yang qi* of a man is not compact, he will contract the evils of the four seasons. However, he may not become ill immediately. Instead, after a latent period, illness develops.

Annotation

[1] The *yin* stores the essence and rises frequently in response to the *yang*: This reveals that the *yin* is the foundation of the *yang*.

[2] The *yang* defends and consolidates the outside for the *yang*: This explains how the *yang* acts for the *yin*.

[3] If the *yin* cannot match the *yang*: The *yin* and *yang* should be kept in balance. If one surpasses another, the balance is lost and both will manifest abnormalities.

[4] When *yang* evils get into the *yang* aspect of the body, one will become mad: When *yang* evils enter the *yang* aspect of the body, this phenomenon is called double-*yang*. The *yang* heat reaches its culmination, so the patient becomes crazed.

[5] When wind evil intrudes upon the body, the *qi* becomes disordered, and the *yin* essence becomes dissipated: The wind evil pertains to the *yang*, so if the *yang* is excess, *yin* essence is exhausted as a result.

[6] Intestinal flux: Diarrhea with pus and blood.

4.1.4　Original article

The *yin* essence stems from the five flavors. The five *zang*-organs storing the *yin* essence can be impaired by the five flavors. Therefore, if the flavor is too sour, the liver *qi* will become overwhelming, and the spleen *qi* will be exhausted.[1] If the flavor is too salty, the *qi* of the lumbar vertebrae will be impaired. The muscles will shrivel, and the heart *qi* will be dejected.[2] If the flavor is excessively bitter, the injured heart *qi* will cause palpitation and vexation. The complexion will darken, and the kidney *qi* will lose its balance.[3] If the flavor is excessively sweet, the spleen *qi* will be damp,[4] and the stomach will become distended and full.[5] If the flavor is much too pungent, the sinews will turn flaccid, and the essence and spirit will be endangered.[6] Therefore, men should prudentially concoct the five flavors in order to make the bones sturdy, the sinews lithe, the *qi* and blood flowing, and the muscular striae compact. In this way, the bones, sinews, *qi*, blood and muscular striae derive sustenance through the five flavors. Strictly observing this rule, one will live to his intended ultimate age.

Annotation

[1] If the flavor is too sour, the liver *qi* will become overwhelming, and the spleen *qi* will be exhausted: Wood can curb soil. If the liver *qi* is overwhelming, it will override the spleen to exhaust its *qi*.

[2] If the flavor is too salty, the *qi* of the lumbar vertebrae will be impaired. The muscles will shrivel, and the heart *qi* will be dejected: Soil can curb water. On the other hand, water can insult soil as well. Consuming too much salt can damage the kidneys, so the lumbar vertebrae are impaired. The water evil is overwhelming, and it can insult soil, so that the muscles shrivel. The water evil devastates the heart upward, so its upward movement causes the heart *qi* to be dejected.

We have introduced the concepts of inter-promotion and inter-curb among the five elements in the foregoing chapters. What is inter-insult? With regard to wood, fire, soil, metal and water, soil may insult wood; metal may insult fire; water may insult soil; wood may insult metal; fire may insult water. For example, soil can curb water, but excess water can insult deficient soil.

[3] If the flavor is excessively bitter, the injured heart *qi* will cause palpitation and vexation. The complexion will darken, and the kidney *qi* will lose its balance: Bitterness can damage the heart, so palpitation and vexation occur. Darkness is the color of water. When the heart fire is insufficient, the water will override the fire, so a dark color appears. The fire deficiency makes the water of the kidneys overwhelmingly exuberant, so the kidney *qi* loses its balance.

[4] The spleen *qi* will be damp: It is morbid. The spleen likes dryness and is averse to dampness. The stomach likes dampness and is averse to dryness.

[5] If the flavor is excessively sweet, the spleen *qi* will be damp, and the stomach will become distended and full: Sweet flavor damages the spleen so that it fails to transform dampness. The damp evil obstructs the stomach, so the stomach becomes distended and full.

[6] If the flavor is much too pungent, the sinews will turn flaccid, and the essence and spirit will be endangered: Acrid flavor enters the lungs. Excessively acrid flavor makes the lungs override the liver. The liver dominates the sinews. So, the sinews become flaccid. Acridness can dissipate the *qi*, so the essence and spirit are depleted.

4.2　Forty-sixth Article

Five Variations · The Divine Pivot（excerpt）

Original article

The Emperor asked Shao Yu:[1]"When the hundred diseases occur, they are certain to result from the wind, rain, cold and summer heat. These evils enter the muscular striae through the body hair. They either turn to leave the body, or linger there, or cause wind swellings and perspiration, or induce exhaustion haggardness, or cause chill and fever, or induce lingering impediment, or bring about accumulation and gathering. The varieties of the peculiar evils that permeate and overflow are innumerable. Tell me why. If two people are affected at the same time, one person contracts one kind of disease, while the other catches a different disease. Does the heaven produce many kinds of wind evils with different affects on the human race?"

Shao Yu answered: "The heaven produces the wind evil and offers favoritism to no one. It is just and upright. One who offends the wind will fall ill, and one who shuns the wind will not catch illnesses. It is not that the wind attacks a man but a man offends the wind."

The Emperor asked: "Encountering wind simultaneously, men likewise fall ill simultaneously. Yet why are the diseases different?"

Shao Yu replied: "What a wonderful question! Let's compare this with a logger cutting timber. The logger grinds an ax and a knife and cuts down trees. The wood's texture may be solid or fragile. Solid wood is difficult to chop, and the bark of fragile wood is apt to crack; the knurls may blunt the edge of a sharp ax. There are both a solid part and a fragile part even in the same piece of wood. The solid part is rigid, and the fragile part is vulnerable to injure, let alone different types of wood, different thickness of barks, and different amounts of sap. If trees blossoming and leaving early encounter spring frost and strong winds, the flowers will fall and the leaves will wither. If trees with fragile wood and thin bark suffer long sunlight and a severe drought, the sap of twigs will be reduced, and the leaves will wizen. If trees with thin bark and abundant sap weather many cloudy days and successive rains, the bark will fester and the sap will ooze out. If rigid and fragile trees are buffeted by a sudden storm, the branches will break off and the bare stems will be injured. If rigid and fragile trees suffer autumn frost and gales, the roots will be shaken and the leaves will fall. In these five situations, there are different injuries, let alone men."

The Emperor asked: "What about comparing men with wood?"

Shao Yu answered: "Most of injuries to trees are at their branches, however, rigid and solid branches are free from being injured. Common diseases of men are also due to the fragility of the joints, skin and muscular striae. The evils lodge there, and the patient endures protracted illness."

Commentary

This section cites an example to describe different textures of wood so as to explain the differences in strength and weakness of the human constitution. Trees with fragile texture are easily harmed. Men with fragile constitutions are apt to fall ill. Whether a man would be ill or not is determined by the strength or weakness of his constitution. To a great extent, a different constitution is inclined to be affected by a certain evil or certain evils. These ideas lay the theoretical foundation for the theory of constitution described in TCM.

Annotation

[1] Shao Yu: A well-known doctor in ancient times.

4.3   Sixty-sixth Article

The Beginning of the Hundred Diseases · The Divine Pivot

4.3.1   Original article

The Emperor asked Uncle Qi: "The hundred diseases all begin due to wind, rain, cold, summer heat, cold-dampness, joy and anger. Intemperate joy and anger injure the *zang*-organs. Wind and rain damage the upper part, while cold-dampness injures the lower part. The three types of evils injure different parts of the body. Tell me about the injured parts."

Uncle Qi answered: "The three types of evils are different. Diseases begin from the *yin* or the *yang*.[1] Let me remark upon the regularity. The intemperate joy and anger impair the *zang*-organs. Due to this impairment of the *zang*-organs, diseases emanate from the *yin*. Cold-dampness assails the weak part of the body, so diseases arise from the lower part. Wind and rain assail the weak part, so diseases occur in the upper part. These are called the evils of three different parts. The permeating and overflowing of evils are countless."

Commentary

This paragraph is a general guideline for the following articles. It proposes the concept of three types of evils, which assail different parts of the body.

Annotation

[1] The *yin* or the *yang*: i.e., the viscera or the superficies.

4.3.2   Original article

The Emperor said: "Of course, I cannot count every one of these permeations and overflows. So, I ask you for the pertinent details."

Uncle Qi continued: "If the wind, rain, cold and heat cannot encounter the deficiency of the patient's right *qi*, the evils would do no harm. One who is caught in a gale or a rainstorm yet does not get ill has no deficiency of the right *qi*, so the evils cannot hurt him. The evils must combine with the deficiency of the right *qi*; the combination of the deficiency and the evils can then settle in the body. When the climate is normal and the right *qi* is harmonious, the body's muscles are strong enough to resist evils. When one suffers due to evils, it is because the abnormal climate combines forces with the deficiency of the right *qi*. This combination produces a harmful disease. Evils prefer certain areas of the body to settle. According to the settling loci, the human body is divided into three parts, i.e., the upper part, the middle part, and the lower part.[1]

"Therefore, the evils invade the body, beginning at the skin. The skin is loose and the muscular striae open. The evils penetrate past the body hair to sink deeper. The body hair becomes erect, and chills ensue, so the skin becomes aching. If the evils linger instead of leaving, they then dwell in the network-channels. When the evils are at the network-channels, intermittent pains occur in the muscles. Then the main channels replace to suffer evils. Lingering instead of leaving, the evils travel to dwell in the channels. When the evils are in the channels, chills with panic occur. Lingering instead of leaving, the evils travel to the transport channel[2] (i.e., the foot greater-*yang* bladder channel). When the evils are at the transport channel, the *qi* of the six channels cannot reach the four limbs. The limbs become sore, and the waist and spine stiffen.

"Lingering instead of leaving, the evils are transmitted to settle at the hiddenpenetrating channel.[3] When the evils are at the hidden penetrating channel, the body becomes burdensome, heavy and aching. If the evils persist in lingering, they will make their way to the intestines and stomach. If the evils are in the intestines and stomach, the intestines rumble and the abdomen distends. Excessive cold there can cause intestinal rumbling, diarrhea, and indigestion; excessive heat there can cause loose, foul stool. Lingering instead of leaving, the evils are transmitted to dwell outside the intestines and stomach, settle at their wrapping membranes, and lodge at the vessels there. The evils linger there and do not recede, and the disease grows into an accumulation (i.e., lump). The evils dwell at the grandchild network-channels, network-channels, channels, transport channel, hidden penetrating channel, paravertebral sinews, or wrapping membranes of the intestines and stomach whose upper part connects with the sinews of the stomach. The permeating and overflowing of evils are beyond the scope of any detailed discussion."

The Emperor said: "Please go into details about accumulation."

Uncle Qi remarked: "The accumulation settling at the grandchild network-channels moves up and down, and the evils converge there. Rendered floating and slack, the grandchild network-channels fail to restrain the accumulation to a fixed area. So, the water coursing through the intestines and stomach converges and pounds until it gives gurgles audibly. When cold exists there, the abdomen is full and thunders with drawn sense. Frequently, severe pains result.

"The accumulation that settles at the foot bright-*yang* stomach channel is located at the side of the umbilicus. Satiety makes it increase while hunger makes it diminish; the accumulation dwelling at the sinews of the stomach resembles the former. Satiety produces pain and hunger produces calm.[4] The accumulation that lodges at the wrapping membranes of the intestines and stomach aches to draw the sinews of the stomach outside. Satiety renders it calm while hunger causes pain.[5] The accumulation that stays at the hidden penetrating channel moves when palpated. After palpation, the patient feels hot air currents flowing down the two thighs as if hot soup is spilling down. The accumulation dwelling at the paravertebral sinews is behind the intestines. It is visible during hunger, and invisible and rarely perceptible by palpation when sated. The accumulation that is located at the transport channel obstructs this channel. The fluids cannot flow downward, and the skin's pores dry up and clog. These are the common conditions that the evils travel from the exterior to the interior, and from the upper part to the lower part."

The Emperor asked: "How about accumulation from the beginning to its formation?"

Uncle Qi answered: "The invasion of cold incurs the beginning of accumulation, and the *qi* reversal produces accumulation.[6]"

The Emperor asked: "What about the formation course?"

Uncle Qi answered: "The reverse cold *qi* makes the feet ache and move inconveniently. The feet ache, thus the shanks become cold. The shanks become cold, thus the blood and vessels become congealed and uneven. The blood and vessels are congealed and uneven, thus the cold *qi* ascends to get into the intestines and stomach. The cold *qi* enters the intestines and stomach, thus the abdomen is distended. The abdomen is distended, thus the fluids outside the intestines are forced to coagulate and cannot be dispersed. Gradually the accumulation is formed.

"Sudden excessive eating makes the intestines and stomach bloated. In addition, irregular life-style and overexertion may hurt the blood vessels. Damage of the *yang* vessels[7] makes the blood spill outward, and the outward spill induces nosebleed. Damage of the *yin* vessels[8] makes the blood spill inward, and the inward spill induces bloody stool. The vessels of the intestines and stomach are impaired, and the blood spilling outside the intestines encounters the cold existing there. The fluids wrestle with the blood, thus they merge and coagulate and cannot be dismissed. The accumulation is formed at last.

"Abrupt attacks of exogenous cold and internal injury due to melancholy and anger could make the *qi* ascend conversely. The *qi* ascends conversely, thus the six *yang* channels become impeded and the *yang qi* fails to move. The congealed blood is wrapped and cannot be dismissed, and the fluids are coagulative. They settle and do not disperse. Then the accumulation is finally formed."

Commentary

This article elucidates three major questions:

1. The article discusses the mechanism of exopathic diseases. It points out that the wind, rain, cold, etc. are necessary conditions under which exopathic diseases occur. The disharmony and deficiency of the right *qi* are internal factors, which decide the occurrence of exopathic diseases. TCM emphasizes the internal causes and the leading role of the right *qi*. The common invasion route of evils is from the exterior to the interior, yet the modes of transmission are diverse and incalculable.

2. The article enumerates many kinds of accumulations that are located at different places and have differing signs. This idea has certain directions for clinical syndrome identification.

3. This article points out that the causes of accumulation comprise the exogenous cold, and internal factors, such as improper diet, irregular life-style, overexertion, melancholy, fury, etc. The general pathogenic changes do not exceed the *qi* stagnation, fluid coagulation and blood stasis, whatever causes accumulation. This analysis offered a reference to curing accumulation in later periods of time by methods of rectifying the *qi*, transforming phlegm, excreting dampness and quickening blood circulation.

Annotation

[1] The human body is divided into three parts, i.e., the upper part, the middle part, and the lower part: or the body is transversely separated in three parts, i.e., the exterior, the half-exterior and half-interior, and the interior.

[2] The transport channel: The five *zang*-organs and six *fu*-organs respectively transport their channel *qi* to their transport points on the back. Every organ has a transport point, which is located on the foot greater-*yang* bladder channel.

[3] The hidden penetrating channel: A part of the penetrating channel, which runs and hides in the spinal column.

[4] The accumulation dwelling at the sinews of the stomach resembles the former. Satiety produces pain and hunger produces calm: The sinews of the stomach are in the flesh. Satiety congests the flesh, producing pain. Hunger makes the congestion disappear, so the patient is calm.

[5] The accumulation that lodges at the wrapping membranes of the intestines and stomach aches to draw the sinews of the stomach outside. Satiety renders it calm and hunger causes pain: The pain of the membranes draws the sinews of the stomach outside. When sated, the inside is full and the outside is comfortable, so one is calm. If the reverse is the case, the patient feels pain.

[6] The *qi* reversal produces accumulation: The cold evil ascends adversely. The *qi* is made stagnant. Then accumulation is formed.

[7] The *yang* vessels: Vessels that stay at the exterior and upper part of the body.

[8] The *yin* Vessels: Vessels that stay at the interior and lower part of the body.

4.3.3   Original article

The Emperor asked: "What about diseases that result from the *yin*?[1]"

Uncle Qi answered: "Melancholy and thought may hurt the heart. Double cold[2] may damage the lungs. Resentment and anger may impair the liver. Making love while being drunken and facing wind while sweating may harm the spleen. Overexertion and taking a bath while sweating after making love may spoil the kidneys. These are diseases incurred by the three types of evils.[3]"

The Emperor asked: "Fine! How are they treated?"

Uncle Qi answered: "We should inspect the symptoms to know the internal pathogenic changes. To the surplus and deficiency, supplement what should be supplemented, and drain what should be drained. Do not disobey the time of the heaven. This is the best therapeutic principle."

Commentary

This article describes the diseases that result from the *yin*. It also presents the therapeutic principle to diseases that result from the *yang* and from the *yin*. Among these, the idea of obeying the time of the heaven underlines the therapeutic rule of taking measures in accordance with the time.

Annotation

[1] Diseases that result from the *yin*: Here, emotional frustrations damage the *zang*-organs. The diseases happen from the interior.

[2] Double cold: In this context, cold body and cold drinking water.

[3] These are diseases incurred by the three types of evils: This sentence is the summarization of the three types of evils, which have been discussed in the foregoing article. They are wind and rain that hit the upper part of the body, cold-dampness that hits the lower part of the body, and intemperate joy and anger, etc. that damage the *zang*-organs.

4.4 Fifty-eighth Article

Bandit Wind · The Divine Pivot

Original article

The Emperor asked: "You say that bandit winds and evils hurt men and make men ill. Now, some people hide behind screens and do not go out of houses. Why do they catch diseases suddenly notwithstanding shunning bandit winds and evils?"

Uncle Qi remarked: "It is because they have once been impaired by dampness. The dampness hides in the blood vessels and muscular striae, lingering and not receding. If the patients get injuries due to a fall or a contusion, the stagnated blood will stay inside and will not disperse. Abrupt, immoderate joy and anger, intemperate diet and improper care of cold and warmth could make the muscular striae closed and obstructed. Meanwhile, the patients are exposed to wind-cold evil. Then, the blood and *qi* become coagulative. The wind-cold evil and the former evils[1] blend, then cold impediment ensues. If those who are sweating due to heat encounter the wind, though they have not met the bandit winds and evils, these people must fall ill due to the combination of the old and new factors.[2]"

The Emperor asked: "Now, all things that you talked about are perceptible by patients. Why does one who has not met evils and has not gotten excessive emotional irritation fall ill suddenly? Is this committed by gods and ghosts?"

Uncle Qi answered: "That is also because one has old evils, which have lingered in the body and have not yet induced illnesses. Thus, when the patient feels repulsion for something or admires something,[3] the blood and *qi* will be thrown into confusion inside. The latent evils wrestle with the emotional frustrations. The disease comes almost imperceptibly and invisibly just like doings of gods and ghosts."

The Emperor asked: "Why could the disease be terminated by a sorcerer?"

Uncle Qi answered: "The sorcerer knows some rules of treatment, and apprehends the source of the disease that demands psychic treatment. So, the disease could be ended by the sorcerer."

Commentary

This article depicts the concept of psychic treatment. It is said that in the primeval times medicine and sorcery were of the same source. However, what is mentioned in the article should belong to contemporary soothing treatment not feudal superstition.

Annotation

[1] The former evils: Here, the evils that have existed inside the body, including dampness, stagnated blood, etc.

[2] If those who are sweating due to heat encounter wind, though they have not met the bandit winds and evils, these people must fall ill due to the combination of the old and new factors: Though the wind here is not an evil, it does induce an externally affected disease. This factor combines with the old evils that have existed inside the body, so one gets ill.

[3] The patient feels repulsion for something or admires something: In this context, emotional frustrations.

4.5   Thirty-ninth Article

Discussion of Enumeration of Pain·
The Plain Questions (excerpt)

Original article

"I know that the hundred diseases result from the disharmony of *qi*. Anger makes the *qi* ascending. Joy makes the *qi* slack. Sorrow makes the *qi* depleted. Fear makes the *qi* descending. Cold makes the *qi* astringent. Heat makes the *qi* discharged. Fright makes the *qi* chaotic. Labor makes the *qi* exhausted. Thought makes the *qi* bound. What diseases will ensue due to these different nine factors? "

Uncle Qi answered: "Anger makes the *qi* ascend adversely, even makes retching of blood and eructation after eating, so the *qi* ascends.[1] Joy makes the *qi* and emotions harmonious, and makes the nutritive *qi* and defensive *qi* free, (but excessive joy makes the heart *qi* slacken,) so the *qi* is slack.[2] Sorrow makes the heart system uneasy. Thus, the lobes of the lungs are lifted. The upper-warmer becomes obstructed. The nutritive *qi* and defensive *qi* cannot be dispersed. The *qi* turns hot inside the chest. So, the *qi* is depleted. Fear makes the kidney essence sink.[3] The sinking obstructs the upper-warmer. The obstruction causes the *qi* to fall. The falling renders the lower-warmer distended. So, the *qi* descends. Cold makes the muscular striae closed and the nutritive *qi* and defensive *qi* stopped, so the *qi* is astringent. Heat makes the muscular striae open, the nutritive *qi* and defensive *qi* unimpeded, and the sweat discharged copiously, so the *qi* is discharged.[4] Fright makes the mind, spirit and thought have nothing to attach to, so the *qi* is chaotic. Labor brings about gasping and sweating, thus the *qi* from the outside and inside escapes,[5] so the *qi* is exhausted. Thought obliges the mind and spirit to concentrate on something excessively. The right *qi* stops and stands still, so the *qi* is bound."

Commentary

This section conveys the idea that all diseases result from the abnormality of the *qi*.

All factors, such as fear, joy, sorrow, fear, cold, heat, fright, labor, thought, etc. must exist under the condition that the disharmony of qi has been incurred, in order to be able to bring about diseases. Meanwhile, the various factors that induce diseases have different features. For example, the ascent of the liver qi shows a series of symptoms characterized by haematemesis (vomiting blood), red face and eyes, a bitter taste in the mouth, sudden deafness, sweating on the head, dizziness, headache, etc. The descent of the kidney qi reveals a series of symptoms marked by pale complexion, distention and fullness of the lower abdomen, diarrhea, enuresis, involuntary emission, turbid leucorrhoea, etc.

Annotation

[1] Anger makes the qi rise adversely, even makes retching of blood and eructation after eating, so the qi ascends: Anger damages the liver. The liver qi ascends adversely and forces the blood to rush upward, so vomiting of blood occurs. The liver overrides the spleen, so belching appears.

[2] Joy makes the qi and emotions harmonious, and makes the nutritive qi and defensive qi free, (but excessive joy makes the heart qi slacken,) so the qi is slack: Joy damages the heart, and sudden joy impairs the heart yang. Joy makes the spirit to be dismissed but not stored. Excessive joy can make the heart qi slack, but normal joy can make the qi and emotions harmonious, and make the nutritive qi and defensive qi free.

[3] Fear makes the kidney essence sink: Uncontrolled fear can damage the kidney essence, and result in soft bones, atrophy disease, qi reversal and frequent seminal emission.

[4] Heat makes the muscular striae open, the nutritive qi and defensive qi unimpeded, and the sweat discharged copiously, so the qi is discharged: The yang qi and yin fluids are all discharged with the sweat.

[5] The qi from the outside and inside escapes: The qi escapes from the outside due to sweating. The qi escapes from the inside due to gasping.

4.6   Seventy-fourth Article

Great Topic on Supreme Truth and Importance ·
The Plain Questions (excerpt)

Original article

The Emperor asked: "Fine. The hundred diseases all result from abnormal variations of the wind, cold, summer heat, dampness, dryness and fire. Medical scriptures say that the surplus should be drained, and the deficiency should be supplemented. I presented these principles to common doctors, but they fail to use them perfectly. I wish these important medical theories to be spread and complied with, and the treatments to be efficacious. It seems as if proficient doctors pluck up thorns and rinse stains. What about this?"

Uncle Qi answered: "Ascertain pathomechanisms and do not miss critical points. That is just so."

The Emperor asked: "What about the pathomechanisms?"

Uncle Qi answered: "All wind with tremor and dizziness is ascribed to the liver. All cold with shrinkage and contracture[1] is ascribed to the kidneys. All *qi* with distention and depression is ascribed to the lungs. All dampness with swelling and fullness is ascribed to the spleen. All heat with daze and cramping is ascribed to the fire. All painful sores are ascribed to the heart. All *qi* reversal,[2] and retention or incontinence of stool and urine are ascribed to the lower part. All atrophy, gasping and vomiting are ascribed to the upper part.

"All lockjaw and shuddering to the point of losing self-control are ascribed to the fire. All cramps and rigid necks are ascribed to the dampness. All *qi* reversal with upward rush is ascribed to the fire.[3] All distending and enlargement of the abdomen are ascribed to the heat. All agitation, mania and abnormal behaviors are ascribed to the fire. All fulminant stiffness is ascribed to the wind. All diseases with sounds, where percussion makes a drum-like sound, are ascribed to the heat. All diseases with putridity, swelling, aching pain, fright and fear are ascribed to the fire. All arch-making spasms[4] and turbid liquid metabolites[5] are ascribed to the heat. All diseases with clear, pure and cold liquid metabolites are ascribed to the cold. All vomiting, sour retching and fulminant diarrhea with tenesmus are ascribed to the heat.

"Therefore, *The Great Importance*[6] says: Do ascertain the pathomechanisms meticulously, and grasp the inner links between signs and pathomechanisms. If it has exogenous evils, we should differentiate what properties the evils possess; if it has no evils, seek for other causes. If it is an excess syndrome, we should explore why the evil is surplus; if it is a deficiency syndrome, inspect why the right *qi* is weak. We must first master the curb rule of the five elements,[7] and dredge the blood and *qi* to make them harmonious, thus the peace will be acquired. That is just so."

Commentary

What are clarified in this section are known as nineteen items of pathomechanisms. The article summarizes ordinary clinical signs from the angle of the five *zang*-organs and six evils, and generalizes basic methods of syndrome identification. The explicit and terse description helps us to identify syndromes with facility in clinical practice.

Amid these nineteen items, there are five pertaining to the five *zang*-organs, twelve pertaining to the six evils (five to the fire, four to the heat, one to the cold, one to the dampness, and one to the wind), one item pertaining to the lower part, and one item to the upper part. In addition to these nineteen items, the medical master, Liu Wangshu living in the Jin-Yuan Period (1115-1368), added another item, which is ascribed to the dryness. It says all unevenness, desiccation, crispness, chapping, and stripping off are ascribed to the dryness.

However, we must highlight that these nineteen items are merely an enumeration of pathomechanisms, and they are incapable of encompassing all of the contents about the theory of pathomechanisms. So, in our study proceedings, we had better try to grope for their essence and avoid superficial, partial stress during concrete applications.

Annotation

[1] Shrinkage and contracture: Signs marked by huddling-up of the body, cramping of sinews, inflexible joints, etc.

[2] *Qi* reversal: In this context, refers to cold *qi* reversal due to the weak *yang* at the lower part of the body, or hot *qi* reversal due to the weak *yin* at the lower part of the body.

[3] All *qi* reversal with upward rush is ascribed to the fire: Vomiting, retching of blood, hiccup, etc.

[4] Arch-making spasms: Spasms that make the body turned aside, the back bent backward, and the body curved.

[5] Liquid metabolites: Sweat, urine, sputum, tears, saliva, leucorrhoea, etc.

⁶ The Great Importance: This book has been lost.

⁷ The curb rules of the five elements: The curb rules of the wind, heat, dampness, dryness and cold in nature; the curb rules of the liver, heart, spleen, lungs and kidneys in the *zang*-organs; and their inner links.

4.7   Forty-fourth Article

A Day Is Divided into Four Times in Accordance with
Heavenly Qi · The Divine Pivot (excerpt)

Original article

The Emperor asked: "The hundred diseases must result from the dryness, dampness, cold, summer heat, wind, rain, indulgent sex, joy, anger,[1] and improper diet and life-style. I know that if evils attack the body, the pulses will manifest their conditions; if the evils enter different *zang*-organs, different names of diseases will be determined. I know this. Nearly all of the hundred diseases are alleviated at dawn, calm in daytime, aggravated at dusk, and worse in the evening. Why is it so? "

Uncle Qi answered: "The *qi* of *yin* and *yang* of the four seasons makes it so."

The Emperor said: "Tell me about the *qi* of the four seasons please."

Uncle Qi remarked: "The spring generation, summer growth, autumn harvest and winter storage are the normality of the seasonal *qi*, and men also correspond to this. When we divide a day into four times, morning is like spring; midday is like summer; dusk is like autumn; midnight is like winter. The *yang qi* of men begins to engender at dawn, meanwhile the evil is weak, so the disease is alleviated at dawn. The *yang qi* grows at midday and the growth can override the evil, so the disease becomes calm. The *yang qi* begins to wane at dusk, meanwhile the evil turns relatively strong, so the disease is aggravated. The *yang qi* enters the *zang*-organs at midnight, while the evil devastates the body solitarily, so the disease is worsened."

The Emperor asked: "Why are there some diseases that are not in accordance with the rule?"

Uncle Qi answered: "Yes. These diseases do not respond to the *yang qi* of the four seasons. The ill *zang*-organ solitarily governs the disease.[2] Therefore, if the five-element attribute of the ill *zang*-organ is curbed by that of the day or time, the disease will be aggravated. If the five-element attribute of the ill *zang*-organ curbs that of the day or time, the disease will be alleviated.[3]"

Commentary

The Medical Classic of the Yellow Emperor regards that the waning and waxing of the *yang qi* of the body vary with those of nature correspondingly. Thereby, we can see some diseases shift their degrees of seriousness in accordance with the changes of the *yang qi* of nature. The patient feels refreshed at dawn and comfortable in daytime, and feels the disease aggravated at dusk and worsened in the evening. This idea sufficiently illustrates the integral thought that men and nature are corresponding. This phenomenon is proved by clinical experiences that many diseases possess the property of being milder in the morning and worse in the evening. Of course, the degree of seriousness of a disease is affected by many factors. It is not that all diseases adhere to this rule, so the article further underscores this notion.

TCM regards that every year, month, day or time has its five-element attribute. About this idea, maybe it is the most complicated part of traditional Chinese medical knowledge, which is elaborately explained in the theory of five movements and six *qi* (climatic factors). The theory is based on the movements of the five elements (wood, fire, soil, metal and water), and the changes of the six climatic factors (wind, cold, heat, dampness, dryness, and fire) to disclose the influences of climatic variations upon living things, especially upon the human race in the world. Now, the newly rising science, called meteorological medicine, researches into the effects caused by climatic changes upon human physiology and pathology. It is attracting more and more concern of researchers over the world. How to exploit this complex theory adequately remains a challenge. In this book, this theory is not discussed.

Annotation

[1] Joy, anger: Refer to disharmonious emotions.

[2] The ill *zang*-organ solitarily governs the disease: The ill *zang*-organ solitarily governs the degree variations of a disease, yet the influence by the seasonal *qi* is not manifested.

[3] If the five-element attribute of the ill *zang*-organ is curbed by that of the day or time, the disease will be aggravated. If the five-element attribute of the ill *zang*-organ curbs that of the day or time, the disease will be alleviated: That is to say, if a disease meets some special days or times, it will correspondingly be alleviated or aggravated. For example, when the liver disease that pertains to wood encounters the S7 or S8 day and B9 (15:00 – 17:00) or B10 (17:00 – 19:00) time that pertain to metal, wood is curbed by metal, so the disease is aggravated. When the liver disease (wood) meets the S5 or S6 day and B5 (7:00 – 9:00), B11 (19:00 – 21:00), B2 (1:00 – 3:00) or B8 (13:00 – 15:00) time that pertain to soil, soil is curbed by wood, so the disease is alleviated.

In ancient times, Chinese people were accustomed to using the combinations of the Ten Heavenly Stems (S1 to S10) and Twelve Earthly Branches (B1 to B12) to record years. The combination of a Stem and a Branch represents a year, such as S1B1, S1B2, S1B3 . . . S2B1, S2B2, S2B3 . . . S3B1, S3B2, S3B3 . . . Therefore, there are sixty couples of combinations in all. Sixty years are a round. In this way, it circles and circles forever. The Twelve Earthly Branches are also applied to record the twenty-four hours in each day. For example, B1 represents 23:00 to 1:00; B2 represents 1:00 to 3:00; B3 represents 3:00 to 5:00 . . . B12 represents 23:00 to 1:00.

4.8　Nineteenth Article

Discussion of Jade Arcana and Genuine Zang-Organs ·
The Plain Questions (excerpt)

Original article

Usually, a *zang*-organ receives the ill *qi* from its son,[1] and transmits the ill *qi* to another organ that this *zang*-organ curbs.[2] If the ill *qi* cannot be transmitted to another organ that this *zang*-organ curbs, this *zang*-organ will transmit the ill *qi* to its mother. When the ill *qi* reaches another organ that this *zang*-organ is curbed by,[3] death comes. The ill *qi* must be transmitted on from a *zang*-organ to another, until it reaches another organ that this *zang*-organ is curbed by, death results. This is disobedient transmission of ill *qi*, which may cause death.

The liver receives the ill *qi* from the heart (son), and transmits it to the spleen. If the ill *qi* cannot be transmitted to the spleen, the ill *qi* will be transmitted to the kidneys (mother). When the ill *qi* reaches the lungs, death results. The heart receives the ill *qi* from the spleen, and transmits it to the lungs. If the ill *qi* cannot be transmitted to the lungs, the ill *qi* will be transmitted to the liver. When the ill *qi* reaches the kidneys, death appears. The spleen receives the ill *qi* from the lungs, and transmits it to the kidneys. If the ill *qi* cannot be transmitted to the kidneys, it will be transmitted to the heart. When the ill *qi* reaches the liver, death ensues.

The lungs receive the ill *qi* from the kidneys, and transmit it to the liver. If the ill *qi* cannot be transmitted to the liver, the ill *qi* will be transmitted to the spleen. When the ill *qi* reaches the heart, death happens. The kidneys receive the ill *qi* from the liver, and transfer it to the heart. If the ill *qi* cannot be transferred to the heart, the ill *qi* will be transferred to the lungs. When the ill *qi* reaches the spleen, death befalls.

These deaths are all due to disobedient transmissions of ill *qi*. If dividing a day into twelve parts that are separately dominated by the five *zang*-organs, we can roughly foresee the death time.[4]

The Emperor said:

The five *zang*-organs are communicating and the transmissions have an order. If a *zang*-organ gets ill, the ill *qi* will be passed to another organ that this *zang*-organ curbs. If the disease is not treated opportunely, in a long time of three or six months, or in a short time of three days or six days, the ill *qi* must have been transmitted through all the five *zang*-organs and death will befall in terms of the law. This is called obedient transmission (which differs from the disobedient transmission)[5].

Hence the saying: Knowing the extremely harmonious pulses, we can see where the disease is from; knowing the extremely disharmonious pulses, we can predict the death time. That is to say, the arrival of the related curb time (year, month, day or time) will induce death.

So, the wind is the chief of the hundred diseases.[6] Now, the wind and cold invade the body and make the body hair erect and the skin's pores closed, thus the stagnation of the *yang qi* produces heat. At this time, we can promote sweating to expel the evils, otherwise the evils will dwell at the channels and make impediment, numbness, swelling and pain. At this time, we can eradicate the evils by hot water bath, hot herb dressing, fire moxibustion and acupuncture. If the disease is not treated, the evils enter the lungs. It is called lung impediment, which is manifested by cough and *qi* ascent.

If the disease is not treated, the evils are transmitted from the lungs to the liver to cause liver impediment. The disease is also called liver *qi* reversal,[7] which is marked by painful rib-sides and immediate vomiting after eating.[8] At this time, we can massage[9] and needle the ear points. If the disease is not treated, the liver transmits the evils to the spleen. The disease name is spleen wind characterized by jaundice,[10] heat in the abdomen, vexation and darkish urine. At this time, massage, drug and bath are applicable. If the disease is not treated, the spleen transmits the evils to the kidneys to cause a disease, which is called hernia and lump.[11] The disease shows irritable heat and pain in the lower abdomen and white and turbid urine. (The real *yin* is lost as if the blood is sucked by parasites,) thus the disease is also named bloodsucker. At this time, massage and medicines can be taken. If the disease is not treated, the kidneys pass the evils to the heart, and the sinews and vessels draw each other and become spasmodic.[12] It is called cramps. At this time, moxibustion and drug will be effective. If the disease is not treated, the patient will die in ten days according to the rule. The kidneys go on to deliver the evils to the heart, and ultimately to the lungs (to end the transmission round). Chills and fevers take place, and the patient will die in three days in accordance with the rule. This is the order of obedient transmission.

However, fulminant diseases do not adhere to this transmission rule, or the transmission is irregular. Anxiety, fear, sorrow, joy, and anger may destroy the transmission order, and the patient will be smitten with a bad disease. Due to joy, the heart *qi* becomes greatly deficient, so the kidneys override the heart. Anger makes the liver override the spleen. Sorrow makes the lungs override the liver. Fear makes the spleen override the kidneys. Anxiety makes the heart override the lungs. This is the reason why the transmission is disordered. A man has five *zang*-organs, and every ill *zang*-organ can transmit the ill *qi* to other four *zang*-organs. Therefore, there are twenty-five kinds of variations in all. Here, transmission is equivalent to overriding.

Commentary

The foregoing two paragraphs summarize the transmissions, changes and prognoses of diseases of the five *zang*-organs according to the rule of curb and promotion of the five elements. Commonly, a disease has two probabilities of transmission. One is called obedient transmission that is according to the route from a *zang*-organ to its curbed *zang*-organ. The other is disobedient transmission that is in terms of the route from the ill son to its mother. However, we should underscore that not all diseases obey this rule inevitably. The prediction of death time mentioned in the article is mainly applied to assess the degree of seriousness, unfavorableness or favorableness of prognosis, and probable survival time. However, it is not absolute.

Annotation

[1] Son: As to wood, fire, soil, metal and water, the preceding is mother and the next is son. For example, soil is metal's mother, while it is fire's son; water is wood's mother, while it is metal's son.

[2] And transmits the ill *qi* to another organ that this *zang*-organ curbs: For example, the liver transmits the ill *qi* to the spleen.

[3] When the ill *qi* reaches another organ that this *zang*-organ is curbed by: For example, the ill *qi* from the liver reaches the lungs.

[4] We can roughly foresee the death time: when the ill *qi* travels from a *zang*-organ to another organ that this *zang*-organ is curbed by.

[5] This is called obedient transmission (which differs from the disobedient transmission): There are two types of transmissions. One is disobedient transmission, and the other is obedient transmis-

sion, which will be further discussed in the following article.

[6] The wind is the chief of the hundred diseases: The wind is the leader of the six evils. It always acts as the leader of exogenous evils to cause diseases.

[7] Liver *qi* reversal: The liver *qi* is liable to ascend in reverse.

[8] Immediate vomiting after eating: The wood (liver) overrides the spleen.

[9] Massage: Massage to resolve the liver stagnation.

[10] Jaundice: The wind and dampness produce heat in the spleen. So, dampness and heat make jaundice.

[11] Hernia and lump: Here refer to lumps in the lower abdomen, which induce pains in the private parts.

[12] The sinews and vessels draw each other and become spasmodic: The heart dominates the blood and vessels. When the heart is impaired, the sinews and vessels will lose their nourishment. So they draw each other and become spasmodic.

Chapter Five
Diseases and Symptoms

The contents that we will discuss in this chapter focus on three categories. The first is disease. A disease is a pathogenic course that has a certain style of manifestation. The occurrence, development, variations, and symptoms of every disease, such as epilepsy, possess distinct regularity. The second is symptom. Symptoms are patients' subjective abnormal feelings and unusual variations inspected by doctors, such as cough, headache, fever, etc. The third is disease group, which is characterized by a major symptom, such as febrile diseases, atrophy diseases, edema, etc.

Diseases and signs are organically classified according to their attributes of pathogens and pathomechanisms, based on the internal injury, exogenous affection, five *zang*-organs, six *fu*-organs, channels, etc. For example, febrile diseases include fevers due to exogenous affection by wind and cold, fevers due to exuberance of the *yin* or *yang* caused by internal emotional injury, etc. Cough signs encompass coughs of the five *zang*-organs and coughs of the six *fu*-organs. *Qi* reversal signs comprise *qi* reversals of the six channels, *qi* reversals of the twelve channels, etc. All these sufficiently reveal the fundamental feature of syndrome identification and treatment determination in TCM.

The Medical Classic of the Yellow Emperor collects more than a hundred different diseases and signs. Some of them are discussed in special articles, and some are intermittently seen in many chapters. *The Medical Classic of the Yellow Emperor* concisely and systematically expatiates upon the pathogen, pathomechanism, clinical symptoms, classification of diagnosis, therapeutic principle and method, prognosis, and prevention of every disease. All such knowledge reflects the people's cognitive abilities with diseases in those archaic times (more than two thousand years ago).

Although it is impossible for these knowledge to be flawless in analysis and understanding, most of its ideas possess authoritative and directive importance even today, and these incisive and scientific descriptions cannot be devalued. Mastering these knowledge will be undoubtedly helpful to improve our levels of both theory and "syndrome identification and treatment determination" of TCM.

Febrile Diseases

5.1   Thirty-first Article

Discussion of Febrile Diseases · The Plain Questions

5.1.1   Original article

The Emperor asked: "Generally, febrile diseases pertain to externally affected diseases. Patients recover or die. The time of death is usually in six or seven days, or the recuperation time is usually more than ten days. Why is it so? Explain this please."

Uncle Qi answered: "All *yang* channels are ascribed to the foot greater-*yang* bladder channel.[1] The foot greater-*yang* bladder channel connects with the *fengfu* point,[2] so it is the chief of all *yang* channels. If a man is impaired by exogenous evils, fever may occur. Even though the fever is high, the patient will not die. If getting dual contraction of evils,[3] the patient will not survive the disease."

The Emperor asked: "What about its condition?"

Uncle Qi answered: "If one contracts exogenous evils on the first day,[4] the foot greater-*yang* bladder channel is attacked. So, the head and neck are painful, and the loins and spine are stiff. On the second day, the foot bright-*yang* stomach channel is attacked. The bright-*yang* dominates the flesh, and its line closely flanks the side of the nose and connects with the eye, so one gets a feverish body, painful eyes, dry nose and sleeplessness. On the third day, the foot lesser-*yang* gallbladder is smitten. The lesser-*yang* channel dominates the gallbladder, and its line goes through the rib-side and connects with the ear, so the chest and rib-sides are painful and deafness occurs. If the three *yang* channels are affected, but the evils have not infringed upon the three *yin* channels, sweating (diaphoresis) can stop the disease.

"On the fourth day, the foot greater-*yin* spleen channel is assailed. Its line is located in the stomach and connects with the throat, so the patient feels the abdomen full and the throat dry. On the fifth day, the foot lesser-*yin* kidney channel is hit. Its line penetrates through the kidney, connects with the lung, and links up with the root of the tongue, so dry mouth and tongue and thirst occur. On the sixth day, the foot cold-*yin* liver channel is assailed. Its line goes around the genitals and connects with the liver, so one feels vexed and depressed, and a man's scrotum shrinks. The three *yin* channels, three *yang* channels, five *zang*-organs, and six *fu*-organs are contaminated. The nutritive *qi* and defensive *qi* do not flow. The five *zang*-organs are obstructed. So the patient will die.

"If one is not dually affected by evils, on the seventh day the disease of the greater-*yang* weakens, and the headache is slightly relieved. On the eighth day, the disease of the bright-*yang* declines, and the fever subsides a little bit. On the ninth day, the disease of the lesser-*yang* is palliated and the deaf ears can hear something. On the tenth day, the disease of the greater-*yin* is alleviated, and the full abdomen returns to its previous state, so one desires food. On the eleventh day, the disease of the lesser-*yin* is mitigated. The thirst is allayed. The dry tongue becomes moist. The patient sneezes. On the twelfth day, the disease of the cold-*yin* weakens, and the shrunken scrotum and lower abdomen become relaxed. The pernicious evils all recede, and the ill course is thereby over."

The Emperor asked: "How are the diseases treated?"

Uncle Qi answered: "Treat to dredge the ill *zang-fu* organs and channels so that the evils weaken and the diseases terminate. For a disease that has not lasted three days, sweating can stop it; for a disease that has lasted three days, draining (heat) can stop it.[5]"

The Emperor asked: "When a febrile disease recovers, there is often a little remnant fever. Why?"

Uncle Qi answered: "All remnant fever is due to forced eating during a high fever, therefore there is a remnant fever. In this way, although the disease weakens, the remnant heat is stored because the fever wrestles with the heat of the food. These two kinds of heat blend, and therefore a remnant fever happens."

The Emperor said: "That is great! How does one treat a remnant fever?"

Uncle Qi answered: "By looking at its excess or deficiency and adjusting its disobedience and obedience, we can stop it."

The Emperor asked: "What is the contraindication of febrile diseases?"

Uncle Qi answered: "When a febrile disease recovers a little, having an appropriate amount of meat will help its rehabilitation,[6] and taking too much meat will incur a remnant fever. That is the contraindication."

Commentary

This article tersely explains the common rule of transmission of exopathogenic febrile diseases, major symptoms of diseased six channels, general therapeutic principle, prognosis, and contraindication. The article enumerates the symptoms of the diseased three *yang* and three *yin* channels, denoting the gist of syndrome identification and transmission process. It points out that this kind of exopathogenic febrile diseases possesses a feature of transmission, i.e., from the exterior to the interior. These explanations formed the theoretical basis for syndrome identification of the six channels in *The Discussion on Damage from Cold*, written by the great medical master, Zhang Zhongjing, who lived in the Eastern Han Dynasty (25-220). However, exopathogenic diseases vary unpredictably, so what we talk about here is merely the routine not specialties.

The therapeutic method of draining described in *The Medical Classic of the Yellow Emperor* mainly refers to acupuncture. In later periods of time, the method of draining was widened and developed to become discharging heat, offensive purgation, diuresis, expelling blood stasis, etc.

Annotation

[1] All *yang* channels are ascribed to the foot greater-*yang* bladder channel: All *yang* channels here refer to the governing channel and *yang*-linking channel. The governing channel, whose major line runs in the spine, is the sea of all *yang* channels. The *yang*-linking channel links up with all *yang* channels. They generally meet at the *fengfu* point, which pertains to the foot greater-*yang* bladder channel. So, the foot greater-*yang* bladder channel is the chief of all *yang* channels.

[2] The *fengfu* point: Also known as GV-16 who (Wind House). It pertains to the governing channel and is located on the median line of the nape, one thumb-width above the hairline.

[3] Dual contraction of evils: An exterior channel and its corresponding interior channel are attacked simultaneously. For example, the foot greater-*yang* bladder channel and foot lesser-*yin* kidney channel are hit at the same time.

[4] The first day: The first day, second day, third day ... sixth day in this context are not definite dates but development stages of febrile diseases.

[5] For a disease that has not lasted three days, sweating can stop it; for a disease that has lasted three days, draining (heat) can stop it: A disease that has not lasted three days is at the three *yang* channels. A disease that has lasted three days is at the three *yin* channels.

[6] Having an appropriate amount of meat will help its rehabilitation: Means taking some nutritious foods.

5.1.2   Original article

The Emperor asked: "If one dually contracts evils, what about his pulse and symptoms?"

Uncle Qi answered: "One is dually hit by evils. On the first day, the foot greater-*yang* bladder channel and foot lesser-*yin* kidney channel become unhealthy simultaneously. Headache, dry mouth and vexation occur. On the second day, the foot bright-*yang* stomach channel and foot greater-*yin* spleen channel fall ill simultaneously. Abdominal fullness, hot body, loss of appetite, and delirium may ensue. On the third day, the foot lesser-*yang* gallbladder channel and foot cold-*yin* liver channel get ill at the same time. Deafness, shrunken scrotum and cold limbs arise. The patient cannot drink water and loses consciousness. On the sixth day, the patient dies."

The Emperor asked: "The five *zang*-organs are impaired. The six *fu*-organs are obstructed. The nutritive *qi* and defensive *qi* do not flow. Why will the patient die in three days after this?"

Uncle Qi answered: "The foot bright-*yang* stomach channel is the chief of the twelve main channels. Its blood and *qi* are copious. So, three days later after the patient has lost his consciousness, its channel *qi* is completely used up, thus the patient dies."

Commentary

A dually affected disease in which two corresponding channels of the interior and the exterior are hit, is of sudden occurrence, quick development, severe degree and unfavorable prognosis amongst exogenous febrile diseases. When a dually affected disease occurs, the exterior symptoms and interior symptoms are manifested at the same time. Then serious symptoms, such as delirium, cold limbs, inability to drink, coma, etc., occur swiftly. This condition accords with actual clinical experiences of some acute febrile diseases.

5.1.3   Original article

Among febrile diseases that are caused by exogenous evils, those occurring before the Summer Solstice Day[1] are produced by warmth evil; those occurring after the Summer Solstice Day are produced by summer-heat evil. The summer-heat evil should be expelled with sweat, so do not stop sweat.

Annotation

[1] The Summer Solstice Day: One of the twenty-four solar terms in Chinese calendar. It is usually June 21 or 22 in every year. This day has the longest time of sunshine in most areas of China.

5.2　Thirty-third Article

Comment on Discussion of Febrile Diseases ·
The Plain Questions (excerpt)

5.2.1　Original article

The Emperor asked: "There is a febrile disease. Its fever usually rises again after sweating. The pulse is restless and rapid and does not calm down after sweating. The patient makes maniac speeches and cannot eat. What is the name of this disease? "

Uncle Qi answered: "This disease is called *yin-yang* intermingling. The intermingling suggests death."

The Emperor said: "Please go on."

Uncle Qi continued: "Sweat of a man stems from grains. Grains produce a man's essential *qi*. The sweating caused by a conflict between the right *qi* and evils in the muscles and bones reveals that the evils are retreating and the right *qi* wins. If the right *qi* wins, the patient must be able to eat and will not return to a fever again. The resumed fever suggests the evils are overwhelming; the sweating indicates the right *qi* is overwhelming. When the fever recurs after sweating, it shows that the evils are prevailing. The inability to eat reveals that the right *qi* has no supplement. The disease caused by the residing evils can make the patient's life collapse quickly.

"So *The Discussion of Fever*[1] says: One whose pulse is still restless and overwhelming after sweating will die. In this case, the pulse does not tally with the sweating. It reveals that the right *qi* cannot override the disease. One's impending death is apparent. Maniac speeches suggest the loss of one's consciousness, which will inevitably lead to death. Now, three fatal symptoms are seen without a slightest chance of survival; although the disease is alleviated a little, the patient must die."

Commentary

This article explains that *yin-yang* intermingling is a kind of serious disease among febrile diseases. The article analyzes the mechanism of strength or weakness of the conflicting evils and right *qi* from sweating, fever and variance of pulse to determine a favorable prognosis or an unfavorable prognosis of a febrile disease. It underscores repeatedly the importance of the stomach *qi* during the course of a febrile disease. These standpoints had directive consequences to the clinical practice and the theory of febrile diseases in later periods of time. Although the disease is alleviated a little, the patient must die. This sentence suggests a serious degree and a bad prognosis, not an absolute death. If drugs are given appropriately, the patient might survive.

Annotation

[1] *The Discussion of Fever*: An ancient book.

5.2.2   Original article

The Emperor asked: "There is a disease characterized by hot body, sweating and vexation. Yet the vexation will not be eased after sweating. What is this disease?"

Uncle Qi answered: "The hot body after sweating is due to wind. The vexation, which will not be eased after sweating, is due to the upward *qi* reversal.[1] Its name is wind *qi* reversal.[2]"

The Emperor said: "Iwould like to hear about it."

Uncle Qi continued: "The foot greater-*yang* bladder channel dominates the exterior, so it contracts the wind evil first. The foot lesser-*yin* kidney channel is its corresponding interior channel. The lesser-*yin* receives the heat and its *qi* follows to ascend reversely, so the following ascending leads to *qi* reversal.[3]"

The Emperor asked: "How is it treated?"

Uncle Qi answered: "Needle the exterior channel and its interior channel,[4] and administer herb soup.[5]"

Commentary

Wind *qi* reversal appears in three different situations in *The Medical Classic of the Yellow Emperor*. *The Discussion of Differentiation of Yin and Yang*, an article in this book, mentions that two kinds of *yang* and one kind of *yin* are ill. This disease is also called wind *qi* reversal, which refers to disorders of the stomach and liver. *The Five Variations*, its another article, describes that one who is liable to suffer from wind *qi* reversal has frequent sweating. His flesh is not solid and the muscular striae are loose. These variant symptoms with a same disease name suggest that *The Medical Classic of the Yellow Emperor* was not written by a single individual. Wind *qi* reversal mentioned in this article pertains to febrile diseases.

Annotation

[1] The upward *qi* reversal: The upward *qi* reversal of the lesser-*yin* kidney channel.

[2] Its name is wind *qi* reversal: Means *qi* reversal due to wind. The foot greater-*yang* bladder channel is affected by wind, and the *qi* of the foot lesser-*yin* kidney channel follows to ascend reversely.

[3] The lesser-*yin* receives the heat and its *qi* follows to ascend reversely, so the following ascending leads to *qi* reversal: The foot greater-*yang* bladder channel is affected and heat is produced. The foot lesser-*yin* kidney channel acts reciprocally with it, so the lesser-*yin* receives the

heat from the greater-*yang* and its *qi* follows to ascend. The evils and the right *qi* conflict at the interior, so the hot body and vexation are not eased after sweating. The interior (lesser-*yin*) and exterior (greater-*yang*) are both ill in this disease.

⁴ Needle the exterior channel and its interior channel: To drain the heat of the greater-*yang* and supplement the deficient *qi* of the lesser-*yin*.

⁵ Administer herb soup: The evils are overwhelming, while the right *qi* is weak. Administer soup to heal the illness.

5.2.3 Original article

The Emperor asked: "What is labor wind disease?"

Uncle Qi answered: "Labor wind disease usually occurs below the lungs.[1] The disease makes the head and neck stiff, and causes dim eyesight. The sputum is like tears. The patient is averse to wind and shudders with cold. This is labor wind disease."

The Emperor asked: "How is it treated?"

Uncle Qi answered: "The doctor should ease up the bending and stretching of the head and neck, and acupuncture the greater-*yang* bladder channel to lead its *qi*. The young men in three days, the middle-aged in five days and the old in seven days, will recover.[2] The patient expectorates blue and yellow sputum like pus in shape and like little balls in volume from the mouth and nose. If he does not, the lungs will be impaired. The impaired lungs may induce death."

Annotation

[1] Labor wind disease usually occurs below the lungs: The patient catches the wind evil because of his deficiency caused by labor. Labor makes the fire rise from below, then the wind evil attacks. The fire and wind wrestle and ascend, so the disease usually occurs below the lungs.

[2] The young men in three days, the middle-aged in five days and the old in seven days, will recover: It refers to approximate time when the disease is alleviated.

5.3 Sixty-first Article

Five Contraindications · The Divine Pivot (*excerpt*)

Original article

The Emperor asked: "What are five unfavorable conditions?"

Uncle Qi answered: "As to a febrile disease with a quiet pulse, if the pulse becomes over-flourishing and restless after sweating, this is the first unfavorableness. If the disease recedes, yet the pulse is still surging and large, this is the second unfavorableness. The fixed impediment does not move. The flesh around big joints is broken. The body is hot. The pulse is almost disappearing. This is the third unfavorableness. As to a licentious man who is haggard, if the body is hot, the color is wan, and feces have much purple and dark stagnant blood, this is the fourth unfavorableness. If chill and fever impair the patient to make him emaciated, and the pulse beats strongly,[1] this is the fifth unfavorableness."

Commentary

This article enunciates the five unfavorable conditions of febrile diseases. These five kinds of signs show that evils are overwhelming, yet the right *qi* is feeble to defend a man from harm. These five conditions all have unfavorable prognoses. In clinical practice, mastering symptoms and pathomechanisms of these five unfavorable conditions is vital to syndrome identification and treatment determination of febrile diseases.

Annotation

[1] Chill and fever impair the patient to make him emaciated, and the pulse beats strongly: It suggests that the spleen *yin* is seriously damaged, thus the pulse of the genuine *zang*-organ (the spleen) is exhibited.

Cough

5.4   Thirty-eighth Article

Discussion of Cough · The Plain Questions

5.4.1   Original article

The Emperor asked: "Why do the lungs make men cough?"

Uncle Qi answered: "The five *zang*-organs and six *fu*-organs can all make men cough, not only the lungs do."

The Emperor said: "I would like to hear about this."

Uncle Qi remarked: "The skin and body hair are the external correspondence to the lungs. The skin and body hair are attacked by evils first, and then the evils enter the lungs. When cold drinks and foods enter the stomach, the cold ascends to the lungs along the blood vessels of the lungs, so the lungs become cold. If the lungs are cold, the external cold and internal cold combine and settle at the lungs, so a lung cough occurs.

"The five *zang*-organs contract evils in their dominated seasons respectively. If it is not autumn, the other four *zang*-organs transfer the evils to the lungs. Man and nature are mutually corresponding, therefore the five *zang*-organs catch the cold and get ill in their dominated seasons respectively. If the disease is slight, it is a cough; if serious, diarrhea and pain may ensue.[1] In autumn, the lungs are attacked first. In spring, the liver is attacked first. In summer, the heart is hit first. In late summer, the spleen is hit first. In winter, the kidneys are assailed first."

Commentary

This article mainly talks about the pathogen and pathomechanism of a cough. The five *zang*-organs and six *fu*-organs can all make men cough. This viewpoint discloses that although coughing is a pathogenic variation of the lungs, the variations of other *zang-fu* organs could also affect the lungs to induce coughing. This theory is based on the integral idea of TCM and has direct consequences for clinical syndrome identification and treatment determination.

Annotation

 [1] If serious, diarrhea and pain may ensue: If the disease is slight, the evils stay at the exterior, so coughing may occur. If the disease is severe, it suggests that the evils stay at the interior, so diarrhea and pain may occur. It denotes that the disease is aggravated.

5.4.2 Original article

The Emperor asked: "How can we distinguish them?"

Uncle Qi replied: "The symptoms of lung cough are coughing, gasping with sounds, and even expectorating blood. The symptoms of heart cough are manifested by coughing with pain in the heart, an indistinct choking sensation in the throat, and even a swollen pharynx and a numb larynx. The symptoms of liver cough are signified by painful lower parts of the rib-sides when coughing, even an incapability of turning the body, and fullness of the rib-sides under the armpits when turning the body. The symptoms of spleen cough are marked by pain at the lower part of the right rib-side when coughing, faint pain radiating to the shoulders and back, even incapability of movement and a more severe cough when moving. The symptoms of kidney cough are characterized by painful loins and back when coughing, and even expectorating saliva and thin sputum."

The Emperor asked: "What about coughs of the six *fu*-organs? How do they receive evils?"

Uncle Qi answered: "The prolonged coughs of the five *zang*-organs may be transmitted to the six *fu*-organs. If spleen cough is not cured, it may affect the stomach. The symptoms of stomach cough are coughing, vomiting, and even retching roundworms in bad vomiting. If liver cough is not cured, it may be transmitted to the gallbladder. Gallbladder cough is marked by coughing and vomiting bile. If lung cough is not cured, it may be passed to the large-intestine. Large-intestine cough is signified by a cough and incontinence of feces. If heart cough is not cured, it may contaminate the small-intestine. Small-intestine cough is characterized by coughing and passing gas. If kidney cough is not cured, it may be transferred to the bladder. The symptoms of bladder cough are a cough and incontinence of urine. If these coughs cannot be stopped for a long time, the triple-warmer will receive disease. Triple-warmer cough is manifested by coughing, abdominal fullness, and no desire for food and drink.

"All these coughs are due to water converging in the stomach, and are relevant to the lungs.[1] They can make the patient have much phlegm, and cause facial edema and *qi* reversal."

Commentary

These two segments discuss the separate symptoms of coughs of the five *zang*-organs and six *fu*-organs. The signs that we see are the main reference to our syndrome identification. This idea offered an example for syndrome identification of the *zang-fu* organs in later periods of time.

This article emphasizes that the lungs and stomach are relevant to the occurrence of a cough. If a cough is endless, it will affect the functioning of the triple-warmer in transforming water, and the fluids will become stagnant and turn into phlegm and rheum. The phlegm and rheum converge at the stomach and attack the lungs upward. So, much sputum, facial edema, and *qi* reversal will occur. Evidently, the theory that the spleen is the source of phlegm, and the lungs are the vessel to store phlegm originate from here.

Annotation

[1] All these coughs are due to water converging in the stomach, and are relevant to the lungs: Though the five *zang*-organs and six *fu*-organs can all make one cough, the stomach and lungs are more intimately pertinent to coughing.

5.4.3 Original article

The Emperor asked: "What about the treatments?"

Uncle Qi answered: "Treat the inrush points[1] to coughs of the *zang*-organs. Treat the entrance points[1] to coughs of the *fu*-organs. Treat the pass points[1] to edema."

The Emperor said: "Magnificent!"

Commentary

This article mentions the general therapeutic principle of acupuncture to cough. It also encompasses the idea of treatment determination according to channel differentiation.

Annotation

[1] The inrush points, entrance points and pass points: There are some specific points below the joints of the elbows and knees, located on the twelve main channels. Every channel has its own five important points, which are the exit point, the slip point, the inrush point, the pass point, and the entrance point. The flow of the channel *qi* seems like waters running in a river. So, the exit point means where the channel *qi* exits. The slip point refers to where the *qi* slips through. The inrush point means where the *qi* rushes in. The pass point refers to where the *qi* passes. The entrance point indicates where the *qi* enters. In clinical practice, there are sixty particular points of this kind that possess distinctive therapeutic roles. Every point has its name. This is elaborately explained in the theory of acupuncture and moxibustion.

Pain

5.5   Thirty-ninth Article

Discussion of Enumeration of Pain ·
The Plain Questions (excerpt)

5.5.1   Original article

The Emperor asked: "I was told that one who is good at talking about the heavenly laws, must know the corresponding rules of the human race; one who is proficient in discussing the ancient times, must know the contemporary verification; one who is shrewd in observing others, must know how to standardize his own behaviors. In this way, the truth will not be confused and the essentials can be held. This is what we call intelligence. Now, I plead with you to help me understand after interrogation, apprehend after observation, and acquire information after pulse-taking and palpation. You can make me learn all these through my personal experience. Would you mind enlightening me and resolving my doubts?"

Uncle Qi bowed twice and said: "What would you ask?"

The Emperor inquired: "I would like to hear about the sudden pains of the five *zang*-organs. What is the reason?"

Uncle Qi replied: "The *qi* and blood of channels run ceaselessly and circle incessantly. Cold evil aggresses on the channels, lingers there, and does not move. If the evil resides outside the channels, the blood will be made scanty there. If it resides inside the channels, the *qi* will be obstructed. So, pains ensue suddenly."

Commentary

This article signifies the general principle of pain. If the cold resides outside the channels, the blood will be made scanty there. If it resides inside the channels, the blood will be obstructed.

5.5.2   Original article

The Emperor asked: "The pain stops suddenly, or the pain is severe and ceaseless, or the pain is drastic and resists pressure, or the pain pauses when being pressed, or the pressure is useless, or the painful place has touchable pulsations, or the pain radiates to the heart and back, or the pain radiates to the rib-sides and lower abdomen, or the abdominal pain radiates to the private parts and hips, or the prolonged pain induces accumulations[1], or the sudden pain induces unconsciousness and the consciousness is regained after a while, or the pain is accompanied by vomiting, or the pain is accompanied by diarrhea, and or the pain coexists with obstruction of feces. All these pains have differing signs. How can we distinguish them?"

Uncle Qi answered: "If the cold resides outside the channels, then the channels become cold. When the channels become cold, they shrink. The shrinkage makes the channels spasmodic, and the spasms radiate to the little blood vessels outside, so the pain occurs abruptly while it ends quickly when being given heat. If the patient is hit by cold repeatedly, the pain will be protracted.

"The cold resides in the channels and wrestles with the hot *qi* (*yang qi*), so the channels become full, and the fullness makes the pain resistant to pressure.

"The cold lingers and the hot *qi* fights against it, so the channels are dilated and the blood and *qi* become disordered. Therefore, the pain is severe and cannot bear pressure.

"The cold lodges between the intestines and stomach and under their wrapping membranes, the blood cannot be dispersed, and the little blood vessels become spasmodic, so the pain occurs. Pressure can disperse the coagulation of the blood and *qi*, so the pain ceases after pressure.

"The cold lodges in the deep channels that go through both sides of the spine, and there deep pressure cannot approach, so the pressure is useless.

"The cold settles in the penetrating channel that passes the *guanyuan* point[2] and gets up along the abdomen, then this channel becomes obstructed due to the settling of the cold. When this channel is obstructed, the *qi* becomes impeded as well, so the pulsations are touchable there.

"The cold settles in the foot greater-*yang* bladder channel and obstructs it. The obstructed channel causes the blood to be deficient. The blood deficiency produces pain. The *qi* of the foot greater-*yang* bladder channel rushes into the heart through the heart transport point,[3] so the pain radiates to the back and heart. Pressure can help the hot *qi* come. When the hot *qi* arrives, the pain ends.

"The cold settles in the foot cold-*yin* liver channel, which connects with the private parts and liver. The cold dwells in this channel, thus the blood becomes stagnant there, and the channel itself becomes spasmodic, so the pain radiates to the rib-sides and lower abdomen.

"The cold resides at the private parts and hips, gets up and approaches the lower abdomen. The stagnated blood below affects the lower abdomen, so the abdominal pain radiates to the private parts and hips.

"The cold resides amid the wrapping membranes of the small-intestine and in the blood of the blood vessels there, then the blood becomes stagnant and is unable to rush into the big channels. The blood and *qi* linger and cannot move ahead, so accumulations appear after a long time.

"The cold resides in the five *zang*-organs, then the *yang qi* ascends adversely and is discharged outward. Whereas the *yin* is obstructed inside, then the *yin* is severed from the *yang* and the sudden pain incurs unconsciousness. If the *yang qi* returns, the consciousness is regained.

"If the cold resides in the intestines and stomach, then the *qi* ascends adversely, so the pain is accompanied by vomiting.

"If the cold resides in the small-intestine, it makes the small-intestine fail to receive and transform food, so the pain is accompanied by diarrhea.

"If the cold resides in the small-intestine and turns hot, then the intestines become painful, and excessive heat and thirst occur. The feces become dry and fail to pass out, so the pain coexists with obstruction of feces."

Annotation

[1] Accumulations: Tumors.

[2] The *guanyuan* point: Also known as CV-4 who (Pass Head). It pertains to the controlling channel, three thumb-widths under the umbilicus directly.

[3] The heart transport point: It pertains to the foot greater-*yang* bladder channel on the back. Every *zang*-organ or *fu*-organ can transport its channel *qi* to the corresponding transport point that is located on the foot greater-*yang* bladder channel.

5.5.3   Original article

The Emperor asked: "What about knowing after interrogation and understanding after observation?"

Uncle Qi answered: "The five *zang*-organs and six *fu*-organs respectively have their definite manifested parts on the face. We can observe the five colors. The yellow color and red color indicate heat. The white color indicates cold. The blue color and dark color reveal pain. This is what is known as understanding after observation."

The Emperor asked: "What is acquiring information after pulse-taking and palpation?"

Uncle Qi answered: "Inspect the assailed channel. Its solidity, stagnated blood or sunken pulse is all touchable.[1]"

The Emperor said: "That is great!"

Commentary

These two segments enumerate fourteen kinds of pains and expatiate upon their clinical symptoms, main points of syndrome identification, pathogens, and pathomechanisms. They point out that the major factor inducing pain is cold evil. Because cold dominates shrinkage and coagulation, and it causes the channels to curl and induces spasms; it affects the running of the *qi* and blood, and causes the *qi* to become stagnant, so that pains occur. Meanwhile, this article also presents that the cold lingers and turns hot, or the cold wrestles with the *yang qi* and the stagnation makes heat. Then, the *qi* and blood become disordered, and the local part is congested, so pains ensue. Though the pathomechanisms of pain are complicated, they never exceed the cold, heat, deficiency and excess.

The conditions of pain, concurrent symptoms, such as liking pressure or refusing pressure, liking warmth or disliking, radiating pain, etc., and multiple inspections, such as interrogation, observation, and pulse-feeling and palpation, canhelp us to differentiate between them. This idea had an extensive influence upon syndrome identification of pains in later ages.

Annotation

[1] Its solidity, stagnated blood or sunken pulse is all touchable: If the local vessels rise or are touchable, this condition pertains to excess. If the local vessels are sunken and soft, it pertains to deficiency.

5.6 Fifty-third Article

Discussion of Pain · The Divine Pivot

Original article

The Emperor asked Shao Yu: "The strength or weakness of the tendons and bones, the solidity or fragility of the muscles, the thickness or thinness of the skin, and the slackness or tightness of the muscular striae, are different to every individual. How is this related to the pains caused by needles, stone needles,[1] and fire moxibustion? The thickness, thinness, solidity or fragility of the intestines and stomach is different as well. How is this related to medicines? Please explain in detail."

Shao Yu answered: "One who has strong bones, weak tendons, soft flesh, and thickskin can endure pains induced by needles and stone needles as well as fire moxibustion."

The Emperor asked: "How can we know if one is able to endure fire moxibustion?"

Shao Yu answered: "One who has black skin and strong bones can endure fire moxibustion."

The Emperor asked: "How can we know if one cannot endure the pains incurred by needles and stone needles?"

Shao Yu answered: "One who has solid flesh and thin skin cannot endure the pains caused by needles and stone needles as well as fire moxibustion."

The Emperor asked: "Although diseases sometimes occur simultaneously, some diseases are easily brought to an end and others are difficult to bring to an end. Why is it so?"

Shao Yu answered: "When contracting diseases simultaneously, those who have mainly heat symptoms are easily cured, and those who have mainly cold symptoms are difficult to cure."

The Emperor asked: "How can we know man's endurance to medicines?"

Shao Yu answered: "One who has strong stomach qi, black skin, large bones and is corpulent, can endure medicines; one who is thin and has weak stomach qi, cannot endure medicines."

Commentary

This section discusses how different constitutions have differing levels of endurance to the pains caused by acupuncture and moxibustion, and have differing levels of endurance to medicines. This description suggests that we should pay attention to different constitutions in clinical treatment, i.e., "different treatments for different individuals."

Those who have mainly heat symptoms are easily cured, and those who have mainly cold symptoms are difficult to cure. This idea enlightens us that different constitutions may show different physical responses to evils. In a general sense, one who has strong qi is often seen with heat and excess symptoms, and one who has weak qi is often seen with cold and deficiency symptoms. The former condition is easy to cure and the next is difficult to cure. The strength or weakness of the constitution not only determines the occurrence, but also decides the development, transmission, and prognosis of a disease.

Annotation

[1] Stone needles: Medical tools used to expel pus and bleed patient in ancient times.

Wind Diseases

5.7   Forty-second Article

Discussion of Wind Diseases · The Plain Questions

Original article

The Emperor asked: "When wind evil attacks people, chills and fevers, or internal heat disease, or internal cold disease, or pestilential wind disease, or local wind diseases, or other wind diseases may occur. The illnesses are dissimilar and they are named differently. Sometimes the evil penetrates the interior to reach the five *zang*-organs and six *fu*-organs. I do not understand the reasons. Explain these please."

Uncle Qi answered: "The wind evil conceals itself within the skin. It cannot move freely inside and cannot escape outwards. Wind tends to run and changes frequently.[1] When the muscular striae are open, one feels cold. When the muscular striae are closed, one feels hot and depressed.[2] The chill makes one decline to eat, and the heat causes the flesh to become emaciated,[3] so the disease makes one have intermittent chills and fevers and not be able to eat. This disease is named chills and fevers.

"If the wind enters the stomach through the bright-*yang* stomach channel, it ascends to the inner canthi. If the person is corpulent, the wind cannot escape outwards, so internal heat disease occurs and his eyes become yellow.[4] If the person is thin, the *yang qi* will escape outwards, and he will feel cold, so internal cold disease occurs and tears get out.[5]

"If the wind enters the greater-*yang* bladder channel, it runs through all transport points, spreads into the muscular striae, and wrestles with the defensive *qi*. The channel becomes obstructed, so this causes the muscles to swell and ulcers are formed. The defensive *qi* becomes slightly coagulative and does not move, thus the muscles become numb. Pestilential wind disease is caused by the wind evil that makes the flourishing *qi* hot and putrid. Its *qi* is unclear, so this breaks the nasal bridge and withers the complexion, and the skin becomes ulcerous. The wind-cold settles in this channel and does not recede. This disease is called pestilential wind.[6]

"If the wind attacks on the S1 and S2 days[7] in spring, liver wind disease will be produced. If the wind attacks on the S3 and S4 days in summer, heart wind disease will be produced. If the wind attacks on the S5 and S6 days in late summer, spleen wind disease will be produced. If the evil attacks on the S7 and S8 days in autumn, lung wind disease will be produced. If the evil attacks on the S9 and S10 days in winter, kidney wind disease will be produced.

"If the wind strikes the transport points of the five zang-organs and six fu-organs, this may produce wind diseases of the zang-fu organs. The evil enters each organ via its entry-gate (transport point), then local wind diseases are produced.

"The wind moves up through the fengfu point.[8] This leads to brain wind disease.[9] The wind enters the eye system. This leads to eye wind disease, and the eyes become cold. The wind attacks after one drinks wine. This leads to leakage wind disease.[10] The wind attacks when one is sweating while making love. This is known as inner wind disease.[11] The wind assails after washing one's head. This is known as head wind disease.[12]

"The long wind enters the middle-warmer. Intestine wind disease ensues and diarrhea containing undigested foods occurs.[13] The wind stays at the muscular striae of the exterior. This is called discharge wind disease. Therefore, wind is the chief of the hundred diseases. Wind diseases can vary to become other diseases never in a fixed way, whereas the wind evil exists."

The Emperor asked: "What are the differences among wind diseases of the five zang-organs? Tell me their diagnoses and symptoms."

Uncle Qi answered: "The symptoms of lung wind are profuse sweating, aversion to wind, a pallid complexion, frequent coughing and shortness of breath. The disease is palliated in daytime and worsens at night. It can be diagnosed at the area between the two brows,[14] and its color is white.

"The symptoms of heart wind are profuse sweating, aversion to wind, extremely dry lips and tongue, irascibility and a red complexion. When the illness is serious, speech is slow.[15] It can be diagnosed at the tongue, and its color is red.

"Liver wind is characterized by profuse sweating, aversion to wind, a tendency tosorrow, a slightly blue complexion, dry throat and irascibility. A male patient may detest females.[16] It can be diagnosed at the area below the eyes, and its color is blue.

"Spleen wind is marked by profuse sweating, aversion to wind, a lethargic body, disinclination to move the four limbs, a slightly yellow complexion, and poor appetite. It can be diagnosed at the tip of the nose,[17] and its color is yellow.

"Kidney wind is manifested by profuse sweating, aversion to wind, puffy face, back pain, inability to stand upright, a black complexion, and unsatisfied sexual performance. It can be diagnosed at the cheeks, and its color is black.

"Stomach wind is indicated by profuse sweating around the neck, aversion to wind, food and drink unable to move downwards, blockade in the esophagus, a tendency to abdominal fullness, abdominal distention when thinly clad, and diarrhea on eating cold foods. In diagnosis, the body is thin, but the abdomen is large.

"The symptoms of head wind disease are profuse sweating at the head and face, and aversion to wind. The illness worsens the day before wind comes. The head is so painful that the patient is unable to leave the house. On the day when the wind comes, the condition improves slightly.[18]

"The symptoms of leakage wind disease are profuse sweating probably, disliking wearing thin garments usually,[19] sweating while eating, even to the point of generalized sweating,[20] gasping, aversion to wind, frequently clammy clothes, dry mouth, quick thirst and incapability of performing manual tasks.

"The symptoms of discharge wind disease are profuse sweating, discharged sweat wetting the clothes, dry mouth, sweat soakage above the waist, and incapability of performing manual tasks. The whole body aches, and this leads to chills."

The Emperor said: "Wonderful!"

Commentary

These two segments emphasize wind diseases of the *zang-fu* organs, brain wind, eye wind, leakage wind, inner wind, head wind, intestine wind, and discharge wind. They discuss their occurrence, symptoms, and main points of diagnosis. Starting from here, the article enunciates that "wind is the chief of the hundred diseases" and "wind tends to run and changes frequently." Although various kinds of wind diseases affect different areas and have different conditions of occurrence and symptoms, they all possess the same signs, i. e., profuse sweating and aversion to wind. These descriptions clearly reveal the feature of diseases induced by wind evil. They also enlightened syndrome identification of wind diseases in later eras.

All the above wind diseases are incurred by exogenous evils. The "liver wind," "slow spleen wind," "lost heart wind," etc., in later ages referred to functional disorders of the viscera. They pertain to the field of pathomechanism and differ from the concepts that we talk about in this article. The exogenous wind evil induces exopathogenic wind diseases, while functional disorders of the viscera cause endogenous wind diseases.

The article does not talk about the symptoms of brain wind, eye wind, inner wind, and intestine wind. Meanwhile, some descriptions are not quite correct. For example, heart wind has irascibility and liver wind has a tendency to sorrow. Most likely, there are omissions and errors when copying from the original articles.

Annotation

[1] Wind tends to run and changes frequently: It reveals that wind can reach everywhere and there exist so many wind diseases with different symptoms.

[2] When the muscular striae are open, one feels cold. When the muscular striae are closed, one feels hot and depressed: The wind is a *yang* evil. It usually brings heat with it in spring and summer, and brings cold with it in autumn and winter. When it enters the body, the muscular striae are open, so the patient feels cold. The wind damages the defensive *qi*, and prevents the nutritive blood from flowing freely. The stagnation produces heat, and then the heat results in depression.

[3] The chill makes one decline to eat, and the heat causes the flesh to become emaciated: The wind and cold damage the stomach, so the appetite is poor. The heat can scorch the fluids, so the flesh is emaciated.

[4] If the person is corpulent, the wind cannot escape outwards, so internal heat disease occurs and his eyes become yellow: The person is corpulent, and he has compact muscular striae, so the wind evil cannot be expelled. The resulting heat moves up along the foot bright-*yang* channel, causing the eyes to become yellow.

[5] If the person is thin, the *yang qi* will escape outwards, and he will feel cold, so internal cold disease occurs and tears get out: The person is thin and the muscular striae are loose, so the *yang qi* will escape outwards and he will feel cold. When the wind enters, internal cold disease occurs. The foot bright-*yang* channel is deficient and cold, so tears escape.

[6] Pestilential wind: It seems like leprosy nowadays.

[7] S1 and S2 days: In ancient times, people recorded the date with the Ten Heavenly Stems from S1 to S10.

[8] The *fengfu* point: also known as GV-16 who, i.e., Wind House.

[9] Brain wind disease: Its symptoms are dizziness and slight headache when encountering wind, and frequent thin snivel. It resembles nasosinusitis.

[10] Leakage wind disease: Wine is warm and emanating in nature, and tends to open the skin's pores. The patient is struck by wind after drinking wine. The sweat leaks endlessly in every season.

[11] Inner wind disease: The essence is depleted inside and the muscular striae are opened outside. Then wind intrudes, so this is called inner wind disease. The symptoms are characterized by seminal emission, expectorating the blood, night sweat, and steaming sense in the bones.

[12] Head wind disease: Washing the head makes the muscular striae of the head open, then wind enters. So this is called head wind disease.

[13] The long wind enters the middle-warmer. Intestine wind disease ensues and diarrhea containing undigested foods occurs: The long wind denotes the overwhelming wood, which can damage soil. So the middle-warmer is impaired, and the non-transformation of water and grain may occur.

[14] It can be diagnosed at the area between the two brows: Every *zang*-organ or *fu*-organ has its manifested part on the face. The manifested part of the lungs is between the two brows.

[15] When the illness is serious, speech is slow: The heart is opened into the tongue. Inasmuch as the tongue is stiff, the patient is not able to speak fast.

[16] A male patient may detest females: The foot cold-*yin* liver channel surrounds the private parts. If it is strong, one is lustful; if not, one feels repulsion for making love.

[17] It can be diagnosed at the tip of the nose: The tip of the nose pertains to the spleen. The alae of the nose pertain to the stomach.

[18] The illness worsens the day before wind comes. The head is so painful that the patient is unable to leave the house. On the day when the wind comes, the condition improves slightly: The headache in this disease starts or ends capriciously. The coming of wind means the climate changes. The day before the climate changes, the illness worsens. The *yang* evil settles at the *yang* aspect, and the property of the *yang* is early and swift. An early arrival must cause an early retreat, so the disease recovers a little when the climate is changing.

[19] Disliking wearing thin garments usually: The muscular striae are loose and the sweat is copious, so the patient always feels cold.

[20] Generalized sweating: Sweating at the whole body.

Impediment Diseases

5.8   Forty-third Article

Discussion of Impediment Diseases · The Plain Questions

5.8.1   Original article

The Emperor asked: "How do impediment diseases[1] occur?"

Uncle Qi answered: "The wind, cold and damp evils come and mix to induce impediment diseases. When the wind prevails, it is mobile impediment.[2] When the cold prevails, it is aching impediment.[3] When the dampness prevails, it is fixed impediment.[4]"

The Emperor asked: "What are the five kinds of impediment diseases?[5]"

Uncle Qi answered: "Encountering the three evils in winter induces bone impediment; encountering them in spring induces sinew impediment; encountering them in summer induces blood vessel impediment; encountering them in late summer induces flesh impediment; encountering them in autumn induces skin impediment."

The Emperor asked: "How can these impediment diseases move inwards and lodge in the five *zang*-organs and six *fu*-organs?"

Uncle Qi answered: "The five *zang*-organs have their external correspondences. If the diseases are prolonged and do not recede, they may move inwards to lodge at the corresponding *zang*-organs.

"Therefore, if bone impediment is not cured and the patient is attacked by the evils again, the impediment will move inwards to settle at the kidneys. If sinew impediment is not cured and the patient is attacked by the evils again, the impediment will move inwards to settle at the liver. If blood vessel impediment is not cured and the patient is assailed by the evils again, the impediment will move inwards to lodge at the heart. If flesh impediment is not cured and the patient is struck by the evils again, the impediment will move inwards to dwell at the spleen. If skin impediment is not cured and the patient is struck by the evils again, the impediment will move inwards to dwell at the lungs.

"What we call impediment diseases of the viscera are caused by the second attack by the wind, cold and dampness in their designated seasons.

"Impediment may dwell at the five *zang*-organs. Lung impediment is characterized by vexation, fullness, panting and vomiting.

"Heart impediment is characterized by obstructed blood vessels, palpitations when vexed, sudden *qi* ascent and panting, dry throat, frequent hiccup, and the ascending of the chaotic *qi* that leads to fear.

"Liver impediment is marked by fright while sleeping at night, copious drinking, frequent urination, and a bulging abdomen as if pregnant.

"Kidney impediment has a tendency to distention. The coccyx and sacrum substitute for the heels, and the spine substitutes for the head.[6]

"Spleen impediment is manifested by lethargic limbs, coughing, vomiting saliva, and congested upper-warmer.[7]

"Intestine impediment has frequent drinking, obstructed urination, surging and thundering *qi* in the abdomen, and frequent diarrhea containing undigested foods.

"Bladder impediment is characterized by internal pain in the lower abdomen and bladder when pressed as if they are in hot soup, impeded urination, and clear snivel at the upper part of the body.[8]

"As for the *qi* of the five *zang*-organs, quietness retains the spirit while restlessness loses the spirit.[9] Overeating may harm the intestines and stomach. When the *qi* of the *zang*-organs becomes disordered and there is panting, this means the impediment has accumulated at the lungs. When the *qi* is disordered and there are melancholy and thoughts, this means the impediment has accumulated at the heart. When the *qi* is chaotic and there is bedwetting, this means the impediment has accumulated at the kidneys. When the *qi* is chaotic and there is extreme exhaustion, this means the impediment has accumulated at the liver. When the *qi* is disordered and the muscles are emaciated, this means the impediment has accumulated at the spleen.

"If any of the impediment diseases are not cured, they will progress to the inner body. Those in which the wind prevails are easier to cure.[10]"

The Emperor asked: "With impediment diseases, there are those who die, there are those who suffer from chronic pain, or there are those who are easily cured. What are the reasons?"

Uncle Qi answered: "Those whose *zang*-organs are occupied by the evils will die. Those where the evils linger between the sinews and bones will have chronic pain. Those where the evils linger within the skin will be easily cured."

The Emperor asked: "How do they come to dwell at the six *fu*-organs?"

Uncle Qi answered: "Diet and living activities are the root of these diseases. Each of the six *fu*-organs also has its respective transport point.[11] The wind, cold and dampness strike these transport points; and also because of dietetic problems, the evils enter through the transport points to lodge at the *fu*-organs."

The Emperor asked: "How can these diseases be cured with needles?"

Uncle Qi answered: "The five *zang*-organs have their inrush points and the six *fu*-organs have their entrance points.[12] The corresponding parts where a channel passes can manifest the pathogenic variations of this channel. Acupuncture can be administered according to the disordered places so that the illness recovers."

Commentary

This article discusses the pathogenic factors, occurrence, symptoms, treatments and prognoses of impediment diseases of the *zang-fu* organs. Discriminating which organ is affected from the symptoms, can be regarded as an example of syndrome identification of the *zang-fu* organs. The article explains that prolonged impediment diseases of the limbs and body can develop inwards to induce impediment diseases of the *zang-fu* organs, while the original pathogenic factors still remain wind, cold and dampness. On the other hand, the article also claims that "as for the *qi* of the five *zang*-organs, quietness retains the spirit while restlessness loses the spirit" and "overeating may harm the intestines and stomach ... diet and living activities are the root of these diseases." Therefore, we can see that inner factors are critical in the formation of impediment diseases. This standpoint is linked directly to disease prevention.

Annotation

[1] Impediment diseases: The *qi* and blood are impeded in the channels due to wind, cold and damp evils, causing pain and numbness. In some cases, they are equivalent to modern rheumatism.

[2] Mobile impediment: In this disease, the wind is overwhelming. The wind evil tends to run and changes frequently. Running up and down, the pain is mobile.

[3] Aching impediment: In this disease, the cold is overwhelming. Cold is coagulative and ob-

structive in nature, and it tends to damage the *yang qi*. So the coagulation of cold produces un-bearable pain.

[4] Fixed impediment: Its major symptoms are stubbornly numb muscles, heavy limbs, and fixed painful places. The disease is mainly induced by the damp, which is viscous and lingering in nature.

[5] The five kinds of impediment diseases: They are classified in accordance with the affected places. The mobile impediment, aching impediment, and fixed impediment are assorted in terms of the properties of evils.

[6] The coccyx and sacrum substitute for the heels, and the spine substitutes for the head: The feet cannot walk, so the coccyx and sacrum substitute for them to walk. The back is hunched and the head cannot be raised, so the spine is above the head.

[7] Congested upper-warmer: The spleen *qi* nourishes the lungs, and the stomach links up with the pharynx, so the upper-warmer is congested.

[8] Clear snivel at the upper part of the body: The foot greater-*yang* bladder channel ascends to the forehead, intersects at the vertex, and moves inward to connect with the brain. The evil *qi* steams upwards, so clear snivel appears.

[9] As for the *qi* of the five *zang*-organs, quietness retains the spirit while restlessness loses the spirit: If a man is quiet, evils cannot assail. If a man is restless, evils will attack the spirit. So the spirit vanishes.

[10] Those in which the wind prevails are easier to cure: It suggests that mobile impediment is easier to cure than aching impediment and fixed impediment in clinical practice.

[11] Each of the six *fu*-organs also has its respective transport point: On the back, located on the foot greater-*yang* bladder channel, such as the gallbladder transport point, small-intestine transport point, triple-warmer transport point, stomach transport point, etc.

[12] The five *zang*-organs have their inrush points and the six *fu*-organs have their entrance points: In fact, each of the five *zang*-organs and six *fu*-organs has its inrush point and entrance point.

5.8.2 Original article

The Emperor asked: "Can the nutritive *qi* and defensive *qi* also cause impediment diseases?"

Uncle Qi answered: "The nutritive *qi* is the essential *qi* of water and grains. It harmonizes the five *zang*-rgans, spreads in the six *fu*-organs, and then can enter the channels. Therefore the nutritive *qi* runs up and down along the channels, penetrates the five *zang*-organs, and links the six *fu*-organs. The defensive *qi* is the intrepid *qi* of water and grains. It is intrepid, swift and slippery in property, but it cannot enter the channels. Therefore, the defensive *qi* runs within the skin and muscles, steams the membranes,[1] and spreads in the chest and abdomen. If the nutritive *qi* and defensive *qi* become disordered, diseases will occur; if they are not disordered, the illnesses will be cured, and the wind, cold and damp will not assail, so impediment will not ensue."

The Emperor said: "Great! How can you explain why impediment diseases may reveal pain, absence of pain, numbness, cold, heat, dryness, or damp?"

Uncle Qi answered: "These with pain have an abundance of cold. There is cold, thus there is pain. When there is no pain, but there is numbness, the disease has been prolonged and sunken deeply. The running of the nutritive blood and defensive *qi* is restricted, and the channels are vacant, so there is no pain. The skin cannot be nourished, therefore there is numbness. Those who have cold have little *yang qi* and much *yin qi*. This condition increases with the exogenous cold, therefore there is cold. Those who have heat have much *yang qi* and little *yin qi*. The pathogenic evils prevail and the *yang* overrides the *yin*,[2] therefore there is heat impediment. When one sweats profusely and is constantly clammy, this means he has encountered overwhelming damp, and he has insufficient *yang qi* and prevailing *yin qi*. These two pathogenic factors influence each other, therefore there are sweating and clamminess."

The Emperor asked: "How can some impediment diseases be without pain?"

Uncle Qi answered: "Impediment located in the bones causes heaviness.

Impediment located in the blood vessels causes the blood to coagulate and not flow. Impediment located in the tendons causes bending and incapability of stretching. Impediment located in the flesh causes numbness. Impediment located in the skin causes cold. Therefore in all these five conditions, there is no pain. All impediment diseases on encountering cold will be exacerbated, and on encountering heat will be palliated."

The Emperor said: "Bravo!"

Commentary

This article proposes that the occurrence of an impediment disease is determined by two factors. One is the external cause, i.e., the attack of wind, cold, and damp evils. The second is the inner factors, i.e., the disorders and disharmony of the qi of the zang-fu organs and channels. The combination of the two factors can induce disease.

Once impediment diseases occur, the transformation of pathomechanisms of cold, heat, excess and deficiency is decided by the properties of the assailing exogenous evils, especially by the decline or flourishing of the yin and yang of the body. This reveals the significance of the inner factors, and provides a theoretical reference for "different treatments of a same disease."

Annotation

[1] Membranes: The membranes in the muscles and body cavity.

[2] The pathogenic evils prevail and the yang overrides the yin: Those people have overwhelming yang and insufficient yin. When the exogenous evils come to attack, the yin cannot match the yang, therefore heat is produced.

5.9 Twenty-seventh Article

Whole-Body Impediment Diseases · The Divine Pivot

Original article

The Emperor asked Uncle Qi: "When whole-body impediment occurs in the body, its pains move up and down, ascending and descending along the channels. The pains correspond right and left without intervals. Please remark upon the pain. Do the evils stay in the blood vessels, or in the flesh? What makes it so? The pains move so quickly that there is not enough time to apply needles. When the pains congregate at a point, but before a treatment is decided upon, they terminate. Why is this so? Please explain."

Uncle Qi answered: "This disease is multitude impediment, and not whole-body impediment."

The Emperor said: "Tell me about multitude impediment."

Uncle Qi replied: "The pains of multitude impediment occur at fixed places. They can suddenly start and suddenly stop, respond to the left with the right, and respond to the right with the left. But the pains cannot make a complete circle. At times they appear and at times they rest."

The Emperor asked: "Good, and how do the pains occur? Why are they named so?"

Uncle Qi answered: "The wind, cold and dampness settle in the flesh and compress the flesh, making the fluids coagulate to become froth. The froth is affected by cold and condenses. The condensation extrudes the textures of the muscles to make them split. The splitting causes pain. The pain makes the blood to converge. The convergence of the blood produces heat. The heat may release the pain, yet the adverse flow of the *qi* still exists, therefore the *qi* reversal causes another impediment to arise. This is how the pains occur."

The Emperor said: "Great! I have understood this meaning. The evils do not reach the *zang*-organs inside, do not stay within the skin outside, and solely remain in the flesh. The genuine *qi* cannot flow around the body freely, therefore this disease is entitled with multitude impediment."

The Emperor asked: "Very good. And how does one needle this?"

Uncle Qi answered: "When needling this, although the pains have already stopped, one must needle the aching points so as to prevent the pains from recurring."

The Emperor asked: "Fine, and what about whole-body impediment?"

Uncle Qi answered: "The evils of whole-body impediment stay in the blood vessels, moving up and down along the channels. The pains do not correspond right and left. The evils lodge at their places (blood vessels)."

The Emperor asked: "How does one acupuncture it?"

Uncle Qi answered: "When the pains move downwards from above, first acupuncture below them to intercept the evils, then needle above them to eradicate the evils. When the pains move upwards from below, first acupuncture above them to intercept the evils, then needle below them to eradicate the evils.

"Therefore, when needling an impediment, the doctor should first palpate the channels beneath the aching place. Discerning the deficiency or excess, blood stasis, obstruction of the large network-channels, and hollow and sunken channels due to deficiency, he can adjust the channels, or free the channels by pressing warm herb package. If spasms and solidity of a channel are revealed, the doctor should lead the channel *qi* to make it run freely."

The Emperor said: "Magnificent! I have understood them and the treatments involved. Correct applications of the nine kinds of needles should be mastered in treating diseases of the twelve channels."

Commentary

This article discusses multitude impediment, whole-body impediment and the differentiation between the two. Multitude impediment is characterized by pains that correspond right and left. These pains are intermittent. They arise one after another and change swiftly, but do not run around the body. In this disease, the evils remain in the flesh. Whole-body impediment is characterized by evils that stay in the blood vessels. The pains in the tendons and flesh run around the body. Palpation can help us to discern between deficiency and excess. This allows proper therapeutic methods, such as acupuncture or pressing warm herb package, to be adopted. These principles are applicable to a variety of impediment diseases.

Atrophy Diseases

5.10   Forty-fourth Article

Discussion of Atrophy Diseases · The Plain Questions

5.10.1   Original article

The Emperor asked: "Why can the five *zang*-organs make one catch an atrophy disease?"

Uncle Qi answered: "The lungs dominate the skin and body hair of the body. The heart dominates the blood vessels of the body. The liver dominates the sinews and membranes of the body. The spleen governs the flesh of the body. The kidneys govern the bones and marrow of the body.

"So, if the lungs are hot and their lobes are scorched, the skin and body hair will become fragile and dry. If the heat lingers and does not recede, limping atrophy[1] may occur. If the heart *qi* is hot, the *qi* in the lower vessels of the body will ascend adversely, and the lower vessels become feeble. So vessel atrophy may occur. The joints are slack and cannot be lifted as if a broken pivot fails to move. The legs become flaccid and fail to walk at will. If the liver *qi* is hot, the bile will be expelled. The mouth will become bitter, and the sinews and membranes will become desiccated.

"If the sinews and membranes are desiccated, thus the spasms of the sinews are induced, and sinew atrophy may occur. If the spleen *qi* is hot, the stomach will be dry and there will be thirst. The flesh will be numb, and flesh atrophy may occur. If the kidney *qi* is hot, the waist and spine cannot be straightened. The bones will be wizened, and the marrow will be reduced, so bone atrophy may occur."

The Emperor asked: "What do atrophy diseases result from?"

Uncle Qi answered: "The lungs are the leader of the *zang*-organs and the canopy of the heart. If one is not joyful, as if his favorite thing is lost, or one cannot gain what he wants, rough gasping of the lungs may occur. While the gasping occurs, the lungs will be hot and their lobes will be scorched. Hence the saying: Due to the hot lungs and scorched lobes, the five *zang*-organs cause limping atrophy. That is just so. If the sadness is too excessive, the vessels of the pericardium will be obstructed. If the vessels of the pericardium are obstructed, then the *yang qi* will stir inside. Profuse hemorrhage will occur underneath the heart, and bloody urine will frequently appear.

"So *The Basic Diseases*[2] says: The large channels are so vacant that vessel impediment occurs to induce vessel atrophy after transmission. If one has greedy desires but gains nothing, or has many lustful desires and sexual activities, the ancestral sinew[3] will become flaccid, and sinew atrophy will occur with seminal emission or leucorrhoea.

"Therefore, *The Lower Classic*[4] says: Sinew atrophy is engendered from the liver and caused by sexual activities. If one is often soaked in dampness and frequently comes into contact with water, dampness may stay in the body. If the living quarters are humid, and the muscles are saturated by dampness. Then impediment and numbness will occur, thus flesh atrophy will result.

"So *The Lower Classic* says: Flesh atrophy is caught from damp places. If one has a long journey or over-exertion, and encounters a great heat, he will become thirsty. The *yang qi* is too hot to attack the body fluids inward, then the heat may dwell at the kidneys that are the water *zang*-organ. In this condition, water cannot control fire; the bones will wither, and the marrow will become insufficient. Therefore, the legs cannot be controlled by the body, and bone atrophy occurs. Hence *The Lower Classic* says: Bone atrophy results from great heat."

Commentary

These segments discuss the pathogens and pathomechanisms of atrophy diseases. The pathogenic factors of atrophy diseases encompass emotional factors, such as grief, thought, etc., environmental factors, such as climates, dampness of living quarters, etc., and individual factors, such as long journey, over-exertion, sexual activity, etc. These varied factors may cause different atrophy diseases. However, their joint pathomechanism is that the five *zang*-organs have heat. As a result, the fluids, blood and *qi* are consumed inside and fail to nourish the skin, muscles, tendons, vessels, and bones. We can see that the pathomechanisms of atrophy diseases of these five body structures are at the five *zang*-organs, that is to say, the five *zang*-organs can all make people catch atrophy diseases. We should notice that atrophy diseases begin mainly due to internal causes, whereas impediment diseases occur mainly due to external causes.

Annotation

1 Limping atrophy: The disease is marked by atrophy and loss of ability of the four limbs.

2 *The Basic Diseases*: An ancient medical book, which is no longer extant.

3 The ancestral sinew: The genitals.

4 *The Lower Classic*: This medical book has been lost.

5.10.2   Original article

The Emperor asked: "How can we distinguish these conditions?"

Uncle Qi answered: "When the lungs are hot, it is marked by white color and corruptive body hair. When the heart is hot, it is marked by red color and full superficial vessels. When the liver is hot, it is characterized by blue color and withered nails. When the spleen is hot, it is characterized by yellow color and soft flesh. When the kidneys are hot, it is signified by black color and rotten teeth."

Commentary

This article describes the characteristics of atrophy diseases that are caused by the heat of the five *zang*-organs. In order to come to a right diagnosis, we must comprehensively combine them with other symptoms described in the foregoing sections.

5.10.3   Original article

The Emperor asked: "Your remarks seem plausible. But why do medical books say that doctors should exclusively select the bright-*yang* to treat atrophy diseases?[1]"

Uncle Qi answered: "The bright-*yang* stomach is the sea of the five *zang*-organs and six *fu*-organs, and is responsible for nourishing the multitudinous sinews, which govern binding the bones and smoothing the joints. The penetrating channel is the sea of the twelve channels and dominates permeating the large and small muscles; it converges with the bright-*yang* channel at the ancestral sinew where many *yin* channels and *yang* channels gather generally.[2]

"All these channels meet again at the *qichong* point,[3] whereas the bright-*yang* stomach channel plays a leading role. All these channels are related to the girdling channel, and link up with the governing channel by network – channels. So, if the bright-*yang* is insufficient, the ancestral sinew will slacken, and the girdling channel will fail to tighten up. Therefore, the legs may atrophy and become disabled."

The Emperor asked: "How are they treated?"

Uncle Qi answered: "Supplement their slip points, free their inrush points, adjust the deficiency or excess, and coordinate the favorableness and unfavorableness. As for atrophy diseases of the sinews, vessels, bones and flesh, perform acupuncture in accordance with the corresponding dominated seasons of the *zang-fu* organs, then diseases will terminate."

The Emperor said: "Magnificent!"

Commentary

There are three therapeutic principles to atrophy diseases. The first principle is exclusively selecting the bright-*yang* to treat atrophy diseases. Because the bright-*yang* stomach is the sea of the five *zang*-organs and six *fu*-organs, while nine *yin* and *yang* channels converge at the ancestral sinew, and the bright-*yang* plays a leading role. Therefore, except when the method of clearing damp-heat is applied to some atrophy diseases with damp-heat, we ordinarily try to nourish the essence, blood and fluids, and fortify the acquired basis (spleen and stomach) to enrich the nutritious source. In this way, the ancestral sinew can be moistened. The limbs and body can be nourished, and atrophy diseases may be cured. The second is to supplement their slip points, free their inrush points, adjust the deficiency or excess, and coordinate the favorableness and unfavorableness. Under the general guideline of exclusively selecting the bright-*yang*, we must cope with atrophy diseases flexibly in accordance with the concerned *zang-fu* organs and channels. The third is performing acupuncture in accordance with the corresponding dominated seasons of the *zang-fu* organs. This process reveals the rule of taking measures in accordance with time. This idea likely enlightened the therapeutic method in later times, i.e., midnight and midday point selection. (Select acupuncture points according to the running, waxing and waning of the *qi*.)

Annotation

[1] Exclusively select the bright-*yang* to treat atrophy diseases: It means that doctors should mainly treat the bright-*yang* stomach when curing atrophy diseases.

[2] At the ancestral sinew where many *yin* channels and *yang* channels gather generally: The three foot *yin* channels, foot bright-*yang* channel, foot lesser-*yang* channel, penetrating channel, controlling channel, governing channel and *yin*-springing channel — these nine channels converge at the genitals.

[3] The *qichong* point: ST-30 who, i.e., *Qi* Thoroughfare.

Qi Reversal Diseases

(Diseases due to reversals of the *qi*)

5.11 Forty-fifth Article

Discussion of Qi Reversal Diseases · The Plain Questions

5.11.1 Original article

The Emperor asked: "What are cold *qi* reversal and hot *qi* reversal?"

Uncle Qi answered: "If the *yang qi* is feeble in the lower part of the body, cold *qi* reversal may occur. If the *yin qi* is feeble in the lower part of the body, hot *qi* reversal may occur."

The Emperor asked: "Why is the heat of hot *qi* reversal certain to rise from the soles? "

Uncle Qi answered: "The *yang qi* runs at the outer edges of the toes, while the *yin* channels congregate at the soles and converge at their centers. Thus, when the *yang qi* prevails, the soles are hot. "

The Emperor asked: "Why is the cold of cold *qi* reversal certain to rise from the five toes to the knees?"

Uncle Qi answered: "The *yin qi* starts from the inner edges of the five toes, and converges below the knees and gathers above the knees. Thus, when the *yin qi* prevails, the part from the five toes to the knee is cold. The cold is not produced by exogenous cold evil but by internal causes.[1]"

The Emperor asked: "What is the reason for cold *qi* reversal?"

Uncle Qi answered: "The genitals are where the ancestral sinew converges and where the greater-*yin* spleen channel and the bright-*yang* stomach channel gather.[2] There are copious *yang qi* and scant *yin qi* in spring and summer. There are prevailing *yin qi* and declined *yang qi* in autumn and winter. Although the patient has a strong constitution, he is depleted by indulgence in the autumn and winter.[3] So, the lower *qi* is led upwards and cannot return, and seminal emission occurs. Then the evil takes advantage to ascend.[4] The cold stays in the middle-warmer. The *yang qi* becomes feeble and fails to irrigate and nourish the channels. The *yang qi* wanes gradually, while the *yin qi* stands alone, therefore the limbs become cold."

The Emperor asked: "What is the reason for hot *qi* reversal?"

Uncle Qi answered: "When wine enters the stomach, the blood vessels become full, but the channels become deficient.[5] The spleen dominates moving the fluids for the stomach. If the *yin qi* is feeble,[6] then the *yang qi* enters. If the *yang qi* enters, then the stomach is not harmonious. If the stomach is not harmonious, then the essential *qi* of water and grains is exhausted. As a result, the exhausted essential *qi* fails to nourish the four limbs. The patient usually makes love after drunkenness and feasting, then the *qi* of wine and the *qi* of food gather and wrestle in the spleen and cannot disperse. Therefore, the heat prevails in the middle-warmer and is overwhelming in the body. The inside is hot, and urine is reddish. As a result, the *qi* of wine is overwhelming and strong. The kidney *qi* weakens gradually, while the *yang qi* prevails solely, so the limbs turn hot."

Commentary

These two segments discuss the pathogens and pathomechanisms of cold *qi* reversal and hot *qi* reversal. With regard to the pathogens, these two *qi* reversal diseases are produced by internal causes, not by exogenous cold evil or heat evil. *Qi* reversal diseases discussed in this chapter are ascribed to internal injuries. Concerning the pathomechanisms, cold *qi* reversal occurs because the patient indulges in sex or over-exertion in the autumn and winter, and his kidney *yang* is impaired. This condition therefore leads to feeble *yang* and prevailing *yin*. Hot *qi* reversal occurs because intemperate wine drinking or indulgent sexual activities can lead to feeble *yin* and prevailing *yang*. The essential *qi* of the kidneys is closely relevant to both cold *qi* reversal and hot *qi* reversal, though their pathomechanisms are different.

Annotation

[1] The cold is not produced by exogenous cold evil but by internal causes: The *yin qi* prevails, while the *yang qi* is deficient. So the cold starts from within, which is not produced by exogenous cold evil.

[2] The genitals are where the ancestral sinew converges and where the greater-*yin* spleen channel and the bright-*yang* stomach channel gather: Nine channels gather at the genitals. Here, only the spleen channel and stomach channel are mentioned, because the spleen and stomach are the sea of the five *zang*-organs and six *fu*-organs, and they also govern moistening the ancestral sinew.

[3] He is depleted by indulgence in the autumn and winter: The patient was so confident of his

vigor that he did not care for preserving it. By indulging in sex or over-exertion, the essential *qi* was deprived.

[4] Seminal emission occurs. Then the evil takes advantage to ascend: The semen is discharged downward, so the cold evil takes advantage at this weak point to move up to the middle-warmer, causing the *yang qi* to decline day after day.

[5] When wine enters the stomach, the blood vessels become full, but the channels become deficient: Wine makes the defensive *yang* run to the skin first, so the blood vessels are filled first, causing the channels to become deficient.

[6] The *yin qi* is feeble: Because of excessive drinking, the heat of wine damages the *yin*. So the *yin qi* is feeble.

5.11.2   Original article

The Emperor asked: "Some *qi* reversal diseases make one's abdomen full, or some make one suddenly faint and the patient regains consciousness after a half day or a day. Why is this so?"

Uncle Qi answered: "When the *yin qi* is exuberant at the upper part of the body, the *yang qi* will be deficient at the lower part of the body. Then abdominal fullness may occur due to the deficiency. When the *yang qi* is exuberant at the upper part of the body, the lower *qi* will ascend to cause *qi* reversal. The *qi* reversal causes chaos with the *yang qi*. The patient may lose his consciousness due to the chaotic *yang qi*."

Commentary

This article points out that *qi* reversal diseases also encompass a kind of diseases with sudden loss of consciousness (coma). This type of coma is transient and reversible, yet in some serious cases, it will cause deaths. The probable pathomechanisms of these diseases are the ascent of the *qi* and blood, disordered *qi*, and failure of *qi* descent. Just as *The Discussion of Adjusting Channels*, an article in *The Plain Questions*, says: The blood and *qi* run upwards together. A great *qi* reversal occurs to induce sudden death. If the *qi* returns, the consciousness will be regained, or else death will be impending.

5.11.3   Original article

The Emperor said: "That is great! Well, I wish to hear about the symptoms of *qi* reversal diseases of the six foot channels."

Uncle Qi replied: "*Qi* reversal disease of the foot greater-*yang* bladder channel is characterized by a swollen and heavy head, inability to run, dizziness, and fainting.[1]

"*Qi* reversal of the bright-*yang* stomach channel is characterized by mania,[2] wanting to run and shout, abdominal fullness, inability to lie, a red and hot face, hallucinated vision, and insane speeches.

"*Qi* reversal of the lesser-*yang* gallbladder channel is characterized by sudden deafness, swollen and hot cheeks, painful rib-sides, and inability to move the shanks.[3]

"*Qi* reversal of the greater-*yin* spleen channel is marked by abdominal fullness and distention, obstructed stool, no desire for food, vomiting after eating, and inability to sleep.[4]

"*Qi* reversal of the lesser-*yin* kidney channel is marked by a dry mouth, reddish urine, abdominal fullness, and pain in the heart.[5]

"*Qi* reversal of the cold-*yin* liver channel is marked by swollen and painful lower abdomen, abdominal distention, inhibited menstruation and urination, liking bending the knees when lying down, shrunken and swollen genitals, and hot inner sides of the shanks.[6]

Drain what is excessive. Supplement what is deficient. When a channel gets ill itself without being affected by other channels, use this channel.[7]

"Symptoms of *qi* reversal of the foot greater-*yin* spleen channel are tense spasms of the shanks, and pain in the heart radiating to the abdomen.[8] Treat the chief disordered channel.

"Symptoms of *qi* reversal of the foot lesser-*yin* kidney channel are deficient fullness, vomiting, and diarrhea containing undigested foods.[9] Treat the chief disordered channel.

"*Qi* reversal of the foot cold-*yin* liver channel is manifested by spasmodic and painful waist, deficient fullness, obstructed urine and delirium.[10] Treat the chief disordered channel.

"When the *qi* of the three *yin* channels is all reverse, the patient cannot discharge stool and urine, and the extremities become cold. So the patient will die in three days.[11]

"*Qi* reversal of the foot greater-*yang* bladder channel is signified by backward or forward collapsing in a faint, retching of blood, and liability to nosebleed.[12] Treat the major diseased channel.

"*Qi* reversal of the foot lesser-*yang* gallbladder channel is signified by inflexible joints, inability to move the back, and incapability of turning the neck. When intestinal ulcer occurs, it is incurable. When there is fright, death is inevitable.[13]

"*Qi* reversal of the foot bright-*yang* stomach channel is shown by gasping, coughing, a hot body, a tendency to fright, nosebleed, and retching of blood.[14]

"*Qi* reversal of the hand greater-*yin* lung channel is manifested by deficient fullness, coughing, and a tendency to vomit froth. Treat the chief disordered channel.

"*Qi* reversals of the hand cold-*yin* pericardium channel and lesser-*yin* heart channel are manifested by pains in the heart radiating to the throat. When the body is hot, it is incurable.

"*Qi* reversal of the hand greater-*yang* small-intestine channel is manifested by deafness, shedding tears, inability to turn the neck, and incapability of bending the back.[15] Treat the chief unhealthy channels.

"*Qi* reversals of the hand bright-*yang* large-intestine channel and lesser-*yang* triple-warmer channel are denoted by a numb and swollen throat, and convulsion.[16] Treat the major unhealthy channels."

Commentary

These three segments expatiate upon *qi* reversal diseases of the twelve main channels among which there are cold syndromes (or signs), heat syndromes, deficiency syndromes, or excess syndromes. To compare with clinical practice, *qi* reversal of the foot greater-*yang* bladder channel resembles apoplexy. *Qi* reversal of the foot bright-*yang* stomach channel resembles hot *qi* reversal during febrile diseases. *Qi* reversal of the foot greater-*yin* spleen channel resembles *qi* reversal due to food accumulation. *Qi* reversal of the foot lesser-*yin* kidney channel is similar to *qi* reversal due to prostration after vomiting and diarrhea. Great loss of blood, such as nosebleed and retching of blood, could induce great *qi* reversal (coma). Heart pain radiating to the throat and heart pain radiating to the abdomen can be displayed in *qi* reversal diseases of the heart and stomach. All discussions of the original article are not groundless.

Concerning the treatment, the article proposes many therapeutic principles, for example, drain what is excessive; supplement what is deficient; when a channel gets ill itself without being affected by other channels, use this channel; treat the major disordered channel, and so on. We should properly discriminate between the deficiency and excess, supplement or drain appropriately, and determine treatments in accordance with different channels. Serious *qi* reversal (coma) could be treated by acupuncture, which ordinarily brings satisfactory effects except for some irreversible cases.

The descriptions of *qi* reversals of the six foot channels in the second segment and the third segment are not identical. So, it proofs that *The Medical Classic of the Yellow Emperor* is not written by a single individual.

Annotation

[1] Dizziness, and fainting: The excess of the upper part and the deficiency of the lower part may lead to dizziness and fainting.

[2] Mania: The heat of the stomach channel enters the *fu*-organ, and the yang evil is overabundant, thus the patient becomes mad.

[3] *Qi* reversal of the lesser-*yang* gallbladder channel is characterized by sudden deafness, swollen and hot cheeks, painful rib-sides, and inability to move the shanks: The lesser-*yang* gallbladder channel passes the ear, cheek, rib-side and shank.

[4] Inability to sleep: The spleen dominates conveyance and transformation of food. If disharmony is caused in the stomach, then the unrest makes one unable to sleep.

[5] *Qi* reversal of the lesser-*yin* kidney channel is marked by a dry mouth, reddish urine, abdominal fullness, and pain in the heart: The lesser-*yin* kidney channel extends through both sides of the root of the tongue along the throat. So, when the channel is hot, the mouth is dry. When the heat is passed to the bladder, urine becomes reddish. The anus is not free, so the abdomen becomes full. The kidney channel rushes into the heart, so there is pain in the heart.

[6] *Qi* reversal of the cold-*yin* liver channel is marked by swollen and painful lower abdomen, abdominal distention, inhibited menstruation and urination, liking bending the knees when lying down, shrunken and swollen genitals, and hot inner sides of the shanks: The liver channel reaches the lower abdomen. So, when the heat is stagnant, the lower abdomen becomes swollen and painful. The stagnated wood overrides the soil, so the abdomen is distended. The heat cannot be discharged, so urination is obstructed. The *qi* of the sinews is not relaxed, so the patient likes to lie down with the knees bent. The liver channel gets around the private parts, so the genitals become swollen and shrunken due to the stagnated heat. The channel moves up from the medial malleollus to the inner face of the knee, so the inner faces of the shanks become hot.

[7] When a channel gets ill itself without being affected by other channels, use this channel: It means that the excesses or deficiencies of other channels do not affect this channel. We can needle this channel to adjust it.

[8] Tense spasms of the shanks, and pain in the heart radiating to the abdomen: The greater-

yin spleen channel passes the shank and rushes into the heart from the abdomen.

[9] Symptoms of *qi* reversal of the foot lesser-*yin* kidney channel are deficient fullness, vomiting, and diarrhea containing undigested foods: The kidney *yang* is deficient and fails to warm the middle-warmer, so the *qi* there cannot move, and the abdomen becomes deficiently full. The cold attacks the stomach, so vomiting occurs. The kidney *yang* fails to warm the spleen, thus there is diarrhea containing undigested foods.

[10] *Qi* reversal of the foot cold-*yin* liver channel is manifested by spasmodic and painful waist, deficient fullness, obstructed urine and delirium: The liver channel governs all sinews, so the waist is spasmodic and painful. The wood evil overrides the soil, so the abdomen is deficiently full. The liver channel gets around the genitals, so urination is obstructed. The liver stores the *yang* soul, so delirium occurs.

[11] The patient will die in three days: When *qi* reversal is in the channels, it is curable; in the *zang*-organs, it is intractable. When the *qi* of the three *yin* channels is all reverse, and the *qi* of the *zang*-organs is exhausted, the patient will die.

[12] *Qi* reversal of the foot greater-*yang* bladder channel is signified by backward or forward collapsing in a faint, retching of blood, and liability to nosebleed: The bladder channel crosses at the vertex and gets into the brains, so fainting occurs. The injury due to fall may induce retching of blood or nosebleed.

[13] *Qi* reversal of the foot lesser-*yang* gallbladder channel is signified by inflexible joints, inability to move the back, and incapability of turning the neck. When intestinal ulcer occurs, it is incurable. When there is fright, death is inevitable: The gallbladder corresponds to the sinews. When the sinews are not lithe, the joints will not be flexible and the back and neck will fail to move freely. Intestinal ulcer suggests poison there, so the disease is intractable. Fright indicates that the poison enters the heart, so death is certain.

[14] *Qi* reversal of the foot bright-*yang* stomach channel is shown by gasping, coughing, a hot body, a tendency to fright, nosebleed, and retching of blood: The bright-*yang* stomach channel has copious *qi* and copious blood. When the stomach fire is overwhelming, it rushes to the lungs, so gasping and coughing occur. The heat runs to the three *yang* channels, so the body becomes hot. The fire stirs in nature, so a tendency to fright occurs and all blood is made restless.

[15] Incapability of bending the back: When evils are at the small-intestine, they will affect the genitals that are ascribed to the kidneys, so the back cannot bend.

[16] Convulsion: When these two channels have abundant heat and fire, convulsion will arise.

Swell and Distention

5.12   Fifty-seventh Article

Water Distention · The Divine Pivot

5.12.1   Original article

The Emperor asked Uncle Qi: "How can you differentiate water distention from skin distention, drum distention, intestinal conglomeration, uterine conglomeration and stone water?"

Uncle Qi answered: "When water distention begins, the eyelids swell slightly like when just awakened. The neck pulse[1] beats. An intermittent cough occurs. The genitals and hips experience cold sensations, and the feet swell. When the abdomen becomes enlarged, there has already been water distention. When a doctor presses the abdomen with the hands, the sag rises with the hands as if water is wrapped. These are symptoms of water distention."

The Emperor asked: "How can we diagnose skin distention?"

Uncle Qi answered: "Skin distention is due to hovering cold in the skin. The skin sounds like a drum when tapped, and yet is not solid. The abdomen is enlarged. The body swells overall. The skin is thick. The sag does not rise when the abdomen is pressed. The color of the skin remains unchanged. These are symptoms of skin distention."

"What about drum distention?"

Uncle Qi answered: "The abdomen bloats and the whole body becomes as large as that of those with skin distention. Nevertheless, the color of the skin is bluish and yellow, and the abdominal vessels are prominent like sinews. These are symptoms of drum distention."

Commentary

This article describes the major features of water distention, skin distention and drum distention, and the differentiations among them. When we press the patient's abdomen, if the sag rises at once with the hands as if water is wrapped, meanwhile, the wave motion can be felt. This condition is an indication that there is water in the abdominal cavity. If no wave motion can be perceived, and the abdomen sounds like a drum and the color of the skin is normal, this condition suggests that there is gas in it, but there is no water. Skin distention is marked by a swollen body, thick skin, and sag's failure to rise after pressure. Drum distention is marked by a swollen body, an enlarged abdomen, bluish and yellow skin, and prominent vessels on the abdomen.

Annotation

[1] The neck pulse: The *renying* (ST-9 who, i. e., Man's Prognosis) pulse beside the Adam's apple.

5.12.2   Original article

"What about intestinal conglomeration?[1]"

Uncle Qi answered: "Cold dwells outside the intestines, wrestling with the defensive *qi*. So, the right *qi* fails to move normally and attaches to somewhere. The *qi* accumulates and settles inside, then noxious *qi* is produced, and intestinal conglomeration occurs. In the beginning, it is the size of an egg of chicken, then it grows gradually. When formed, it looks like a pregnant woman. After more than a year, it is solid when pressed and movable when pushed, and the menstruation is regular. These are its symptoms."

"What about uterine conglomeration?"

Uncle Qi answered: "Uterine conglomeration grows in the womb. The cold dwells at the cervix to make it obstructed. The *qi* becomes impeded. Malign blood that should be discharged cannot be discharged. Then the congested blood lingers and grows day after day. It is like being pregnant. The menstruation is irregular. Only women can be afflicted with this disease. Doctors can discharge it by leading down.[2]"

Commentary

This article helps us differentiate intestinal conglomeration from uterine conglomeration. The major signs of both are tumors in the abdomen. Intestinal conglomeration is located outside the intestines, whereas uterine conglomeration is located at the womb. The next disease can only befall females, while the menstruation is irregular.

Annotation

[1] Intestinal conglomeration: This disease is characterized by tumors occurring outside the intestines like mushrooms.

[2] Discharge it by leading down: Such as leading method of needle, expelling the stagnated blood, or seating in drug soup.

5.12.3   Original article

The Emperor asked: "Could we use needles for skin distention and drum distention?"

Uncle Qi answered: "First use needles to discharge the prominent vessels on the abdomen, then adjust the channels.[1] Finally, needle to eliminate the prominent vessels."

Annotation

[1] First use needles to discharge the prominent vessels, then adjust the channels: No matter how deficient or excessive, we must first needle to discharge the prominent vessels on the abdomen, then regulate the channels in accordance with the deficiency or excess.

5.13   Sixty-first Article

Discussion of Water and Heat Points·
The Plain Questions (excerpt)

Original article

The Emperor asked: "Why does the foot lesser-*yin* kidney channel dominate the kidneys? Why do the kidneys dominate water?"

Uncle Qi answered: "The kidneys are the extreme *yin* in which water prevails.[1] The hand greater-*yin* lung channel dominates the lungs, and the foot lesser-*yin* channel prevails in winter. So, the root (fundamental) cause consists in the kidneys, and the tip (secondary) cause consists in the lungs. Both the *zang*-organs can accumulate water.[2]"

The Emperor asked: "Why can the kidneys accumulate water and induce edema diseases?"

Uncle Qi answered: "The kidneys are the pass of the stomach.[3] When the pass is inhibited, the water gathers to induce edema diseases. The water seeps up and down along the skin, so the skin becomes edematous. The edema is due to water accumulation that induces diseases."

The Emperor asked: "Does all edema result from the kidneys?"

Uncle Qi answered: "The kidneys are a *yin zang*-organ. The earthly *qi* ascends like the steaming action of the kidneys.[4] Then, the water is produced, so the kidneys are called the extreme *yin*. Gallantry and hard work may induce perspiration governed by the kidneys. When perspiration encounters the wind, the water cannot be stored in the *zang-fu* organs inside, and cannot escape out of the skin. The water dwells at the pores of the skin and runs along the skin. So the skin becomes edematous. The disease is rooted in the kidneys and is called wind edema disease.[5] The skin's pores are also called the sweat pores."

Commentary

This section depicts the pathomechanism of edema diseases, which are intimately related to the lungs and kidneys. These descriptions laid a theoretical basis for treatment determination and syndrome identification of edema in later ages. The root cause consists in the kidneys and the tip cause consists in the lungs. Upon this, the famous master, Zhang Jiebin developed this idea and added that the controlling cause consists in the spleen. The theory that the lungs, kidneys and spleen jointly supervise the metabolism of water reaches its perfection.

Annotation

[1] The kidneys are the extreme *yin* in which water prevails: When winter comes, it is extremely cold; and winter corresponds to the kidneys, while water is dominated by winter.

[2] The root (fundamental) cause consists in the kidneys, and the tip (secondary) cause consists in the lungs. Both the *zang*-organs can accumulate water: When the kidney *qi* ascends adversely, water lodges in the lungs.

[3] The kidneys are the pass of the stomach: The kidneys dominate the lower-warmer and are opened into the lower two orifices. After water and grains enter the stomach, the clear part is discharged from the anterior lower orifice, and the turbid part is discharged from the posterior lower orifice. When the kidneys are strong enough to transform the *qi*, the two orifices will function normally, or they will be obstructed or become incontinent.

[4] The earthly *qi* ascends like the steaming action of the kidneys: The body water of a man is steamed by the kidney *qi* to ascend as if the earthly *qi* ascends to be clouds and then transforms into falling raindrops.

[5] Wind edema disease: Because the edema is due to wind evil.

5.14　Fourteenth Article

Discussion of Soup and Wine · The Plain Questions (excerpt)

Original article

The Emperor asked: "Some edema does not occur through the body hair.[1] The *yang qi* of the five *zang*-organs is obstructed.[2] The fluids fill the body. The *yin* soul resides alone.[3] The essence is solitary inside, and the *qi* is consumed outside.[4] The body does not fit the clothes.[5] The four extremities are swollen and feel uneasy, and the *qi* of the middle-warmer is stirred.[6] So, water is retained inside, and edema is revealed outside. How can we treat this disease?"

Uncle Qi answered: "Balance the *yin* and *yang* in the treatment, eliminate the stagnant and stale water, move the four limbs slightly, wear more clothes, and needle the opposite side,[7] so as to rehabilitate the normal appearance. Open the ghost gate, and cleanse the clear *fu*-organ,[8] then the essence will run normally. Now, the *yang qi* of the five *zang*-organs has spread, and the five *zang*-organs have been tidied up and cleaned up. Therefore, the essence engenders naturally, and the body appearance becomes exuberant naturally. The bones and flesh become strong, and the right *qi* regains its normality."

The Emperor said: "Magnificent!"

Commentary

The pathomechanism of edema is that the *yang qi* of the five *zang*-organs is obstructed and the fluids fail to flow normally. The concerned therapeutic principles and methods are mentioned. All these ideas had a very momentous influence upon syndrome identification and treatment determination of edema in later periods of time. For example, Zhang Zhongjing asserted in his *Synopsis of the Golden Cabinet* that "as to all edema, when it is below the waist, urination should be promoted; when it is above the waist, sweating will restore it."

Annotation

[1] Some edema does not occur through the body hair: The disease is not due to exogenous

evils.

[2] The *yang qi* of the five *zang*-organs is obstructed: The *yang qi* of the five *zang*-organs is obstructed and cannot spread, so the fluids fail to be transformed and gather to become edema.

[3] The *yin* soul resides alone: The *yin* soul pertains to the *yin*. Here, the *yin* soul refers to the fluids and water. Although the body is filled with fluids, the *qi* has left. So the *yin* soul resides alone.

[4] The essence is solitary inside, and the *qi* is consumed outside: There is no *yang qi* in the essence, so the essence is solitary inside. There is no *yang qi* in the *yin* fluids, so the *yang qi* is consumed outside.

[5] The body does not fit the clothes: Due to edema.

[6] The four extremities are swollen and feel uneasy, and the *qi* of the middle-warmer is stirred: The four extremities are the root of all *yang*. When the *yang qi* stands still and does not move, the four limbs become swollen and feel uneasy with edema. The kidneys and lungs are ill, so gasping ensues and the *qi* of the middle-warmer is stirred.

[7] Move the four limbs slightly, wear more clothes, and needle the opposite side: Move the four limbs slightly to help the flow of the *qi*. Wear more clothes to help the *yang qi* at the body surface to expel the congealed *yin*. Needle the right to treat the ill left and needle the left to treat the ill right.

[8] Open the ghost gate, and cleanse the clear *fu*-organ: i.e., diaphoresis and diuresis.

Hot-Organ Diseases

5.15   Forty-seventh Article

Discussion of Strange Diseases · The Plain Questions (excerpt)

5.15.1   Original article

The Emperor asked: "There is a disease with sweet mouth. What is its name?"

Uncle Qi answered: "This is due to upward flow of the five flavors of grains. It is called hot-spleen disease.[1] The five flavors enter the mouth to be stored in the stomach. The spleen moves fluids for the stomach. The stay of the fluids at the spleen induces sweet mouth.[2] This condition is caused by delicious foods. The patient must have taken too many sweet, delicious and fat foods. The fat foods make one's inside hot, and the sweet foods make one's middle-warmer full.[3] So, the hot spleen *qi* overflows upward to induce depletion-thirst disease.[4] It should be treated by eupatorium to eliminate the foul *qi*.[5]"

Commentary

The major symptoms of depletion-thirst disease are large drinking, large intake of food and copious urine. According to its clinical manifestations, it also can be divided into lung depletion-thirst, diaphragm depletion-thirst, middle-warmer depletion-thirst, etc. For example, The Discussion of *Qi* Reversal, an article in *The Plain Questions*, describes that "lung depletion-thirst is marked by one drinking and double urination; it is deadly incurable" and "the heart passes the heat to the lungs to induce diaphragm depletion-thirst." The Discussion of Abdominal Inside, another article in *The Plain Questions*, has that "those who suffer hot inside or middle-warmer depletion-thirst are all wealthy persons."

Hot-spleen disease here is ascribed to middle-warmer depletion-thirst. Because the spleen and stomach are dry and hot, or damp-heat congests the spleen, the fluids are impaired after a long time, and dryness is produced. Its symptoms are large intake of food, a tendency to hunger, haggardness and copious urine.

Annotation

[1] Hot-spleen disease: Disease due to hot spleen *qi*.

[2] The stay of the fluids at the spleen induces sweet mouth: The spleen can move the fluids for

the stomach. The five flavors enter the mouth, then the fluids run respectively in their ways. Now, the fluids fail to be spread to the five *zang*-organs and stay at the spleen only. When the spleen *qi* ascends, a sweet mouth will be resulted in.

[3] The fat foods make one's inside hot, and the sweet foods make one's middle-warmer full: The fat foods render the *yang qi* stagnated and make it fail to spread, so the inside is hot. The sweet foods make the *qi* relaxed and tend to stay, so the middle-warmer is full.

[4] Depletion-thirst disease: Characterized by large drinking, large food intake, and copious urine. It seems like modern diabetes.

[5] It should be treated by eupatorium to eliminate the foul *qi*: It should be treated with eupatorium-like herbs, which have the functions of transforming damp, awakening the spleen, and dispelling foulness by aroma.

5.15.2   Original article

The Emperor asked: "There is a disease with bitter mouth. What is its name? What does it result from?"

Uncle Qi answered: "The disease is called hot-gallbladder disease.[1] The gallbladder is the bilious *fu*-organ that decides the five *zang*-organs, and the throat is commanded by it. This patient is hesitant in thoughts, so the gallbladder *qi* flows upward to make the mouth bitter. Treat the converging point and transport point[2] of the gallbladder as the *Interactions Among the Twelve Yin and Yang Organs* says.[3]"

Annotation

[1] Hot-gallbladder disease: This disease is due to the upward flow of heat of the gallbladder.

[2] Converging point and transport point: Every *zang*-organ or *fu*-organ can transport its *qi* to a certain point on the abdomen, i.e., converging point, and transport its *qi* to a certain point on the back, i.e., transport point. The converging point of the gallbladder is the *riyue* point (GB-24 who, i.e., Sun and Moon) that is located at the seventh intercostal area, three and a half thumb-widths away from the ventro-median line. The transport point of the gallbladder is under the tenth thoracic vertebra, one and a half thumb-widths away from that.

[3] *The Interactions Among the Twelve Yin and Yang Organs*: The book has been lost.

Madness and Mania

5.16 Twenty-second Article

Madness and Mania · The Divine Pivot (excerpt)

5.16.1 Original article

When madness begins, the patient is unpleasant first. The head is heavy and aching. The eyes stare upward and are red. Vexation may occur in serious cases. Doctors should observe the complexion. The hand greater-*yang* small-intestine channel, hand bright-*yang* large-intestine channel and hand greater-*yin* lung channel should be used. He should bleed these channels till the blood color returns to normal, and then the doctor should stop the bleeding.[1]

At the onset of madness, the mouth is twisted, and shouting, gasping and palpitation occur. The doctor should select the hand bright-*yang* large-intestine channel and hand greater-*yang* small-intestine channel. The doctor should attack the right when the left is stiff and attack the left when the right is stiff. Bleed them till the blood color returns to normal, and then stop the bleeding.

When madness is at the point of out-break, the patient gets arched-rigidity[2] first, and the spine is painful. The doctor should use the foot greater-*yang* bladder channel, foot bright-*yang* stomach channel, foot greater-*yin* spleen channel, and hand greater-*yang* small-intestine channel. Bleed them till the blood color returns to normal, and then stop the bleeding.

When treating madness, the doctor should live with the patient,[3] and inspect where he should insert the needles. When the disease arrives, he drains the channels that are in surplus, and puts the bled blood in a gourd. The blood will move when the disease is at the point of onset. If the blood does not move, the doctor should use twenty moxa columns on the sacrum.

Annotation

[1] He should bleed these channels till the blood color returns to normal, and then the doctor should stop the bleeding: When bleeding the channels, in the beginning, the blood is relatively

darkish. When the blood color returns to normal, stop the bleeding.

[2] Arched-rigidity: Equivalent to opisthotonos.

[3] The doctor should live with the patient: So as to observe the situations of onsets.

5.16.2 Original article

Bone madness is marked by swollen and stiff muscles of the gums and cheeks, sweating, vexation and depression. If the patient vomits much saliva and froth, and the *qi* is discharged downward,[1] it will be incurable.

Tendon madness is characterized by a lethargic, spasmodic body and enlarged blood vessels. Doctors should needle the *dazhu* point[2] on the nape of the foot greater-*yang* bladder channel. If the patient vomits much saliva and froth, and the *qi* is discharged downward, the disease will be incurable.

Vessel madness is signified by suddenly falling in a faint, and the blood vessels of the four limbs becoming distended and flaccid. If the vessels are full, bleed them by needles. If the vessels are not full, adopt moxibustion on the points of the foot greater-*yang* bladder channel at both sides of the nape, and on the *daimai* point[3] that is three thumb-widths away from the waist. And also, select all muscles and points that are distended and flaccid. If the patient vomits much saliva and froth, and the *qi* is discharged downward, it will be incurable.

All maniac madness is deadly incurable.

Commentary

This article depicts all various symptoms of madness diseases. According to their symptoms, madness diseases are classified into three sorts, i.e., bone madness, tendon madness and vessel madness. The described symptoms seem like the onset of epilepsy, such as upward-staring and red eyes, shouting, gasping, twisted mouth, opisthotonos, vomiting much saliva and froth, a lethargic and spasmodic body, sudden collapsing to the ground of the body, downward discharge of the *qi*, etc. At the onset of epilepsy, needling is applicable and has a certain effect, yet further research is needed.

Annotation

[1] The *qi* is discharged downward: It refers to symptoms, such as incontinence of urine, stool or gas.

[2] The *dazhu* point: BL-11 who, i.e., Great Shuttle.

[3] The *daimai* point: i.e., GB-26 who (Girdling Vessel). It pertains to the foot lesser-*yang* gallbladder channel. It is level with the umbilicus, just under the end of the eleventh rib. It also pertains to the girdling channel.

5.16.3 Original article

When mania begins, the patient is sad first. Then, he is exultant, irascible, and liable to fear. This condition is due to melancholy and hunger. Treat the hand greater-*yin* lung channel and hand bright-*yang* large-intestine channel. Bleed them till the blood color returns to normal and stop. The foot greater-*yin* spleen channel and foot bright-*yang* stomach channel should be used as well.

When mania begins, the patient wants little sleep and has no hunger. He is self-assertive about his wisdom, eloquence and dignity. The patient scolds and curses unceasingly. Treat the hand bright-*yang* large-intestine channel, hand greater-*yang* small-intestine channel, hand greater-*yin* lung channel, *lianquan* point,[1] and hand lesser-*yin* heart channel. Needle all seemingly exuberant channels, and do not needle the channels that are not exuberant.

Mania with demented speech, fright, a tendency to laugh, liking singing, and endless insane behaviors is due to great fear. Treat the hand bright-*yang* large-intestine channel, hand greater-*yang* small-intestine channel and hand greater-*yin* lung channel.

Mania with visual hallucinations, auditory hallucinations, and a tendency to shouting is due to scant *qi*. Treat the hand greater-*yang* small-intestine channel, hand greater-*yin* lung channel, hand bright-*yang* large-intestine channel, foot greater-*yin* spleen channel, head and cheeks.

Mania with large intake of food, a tendency to seeing ghosts and gods, and secret giggling is due to great rejoicing. Treat the foot greater-*yin* spleen channel, foot greater-*yang* bladder channel and foot bright-*yang* stomach channel, then the hand greater-*yin* lung channel, hand greater-*yang* small-intestine channel and hand bright-*yang* large-intestine channel.

When new mania befalls without the foregoing symptoms, first take the *ququan* point,[2] its left and right, and the exuberant channels. Bleed them; after a while, the disease terminates. If it does not end, needle according to the ways above, and use twenty moxa columns on the sacrum.

Commentary

This article describes varied symptoms of mania diseases, causes and acupuncture point selections. These symptoms are frequently seen in mental diseases. So, it shows that at the times of *The Medical Classic of the Yellow Emperor*, people had learnt psychosis.

Annotation

[1] The *lianquan* point: i.e., CV-23 who (Ridge Spring). It pertains to the controlling channel and is located at the middle point of the upper edge of the hyoid bone.

[2] The *ququan* point: i.e., LV-8 (Curved Spring). It pertains to the foot cold-*yin* liver channel and is located at the inner end of the transverse line of the back of knee.

5.17　Forty-seventh Article

Discussion of Strange Diseases ·
The Plain Questions (excerpt)

Original article

The Emperor asked: "There are some congenital madness diseases. What names do they have? How are they caused?"

Uncle Qi answered: "They are called fetus diseases. A fetus disease is contracted in pregnancy during which the mother suffers from great fear that may induce the *qi* to ascend and not return. The essential *qi* and disordered *qi* blend, so the baby catches a congenital madness disease."

Commentary

This article points out some madness diseases (such as epilepsy, etc.) are due to congenital factors. A woman during pregnancy may be blown by great emotional frustrations, so her baby may catch an inborn disease. This description epitomizes that in early times people had learnt an understanding of the significance of hygiene during gestation. Pregnant women should keep happy, avoid emotional irritations, and take care of antenatal instruction. This idea is also a reflex of assertion about eugenics in *The Medical Classic of the Yellow Emperor*.

5.18 Forty-sixth Article

Discussion of Symptoms · The Plain Questions (*excerpt*)

Original article

The Emperor asked: "There is furious mania. What does it result from?"

Uncle Qi answered: "The disease results from the *yang qi*."

The Emperor asked: "How could the *yang qi* cause one to be maniac?"

Uncle Qi answered: "The *yang qi* is suddenly frustrated by emotional irritations and becomes irresolute and disordered, so the patient becomes irascible. The disease is called *yang qi* reversal."

The Emperor asked: "How can you know this?"

Uncle Qi answered: "The foot bright-*yang* stomach channel has many pulsating points of vessels.[1] The foot greater-*yang* bladder channel and foot lesser-*yang* gallbladder channel nearly have no pulsating points of vessels. However, the two channels become pulsating, large and rapid in this case.[2] These are its symptoms."

The Emperor asked: "How can we treat it?"

Uncle Qi answered: "Force the patient to starve,[3] then the disease will end. Foods enter the *yin*,[4] which produces the *yang qi*. So, if foods are deprived, the disease will terminate without the source of the *yang qi*.[5] The patient should be asked to take the Beverage of Raw Iron Powders, which can lower the *qi* swiftly.[6]"

Annotation

[1] The foot bright-*yang* stomach channel has many pulsating points of vessels: Such as the *chongyang* point (ST-42 who, i.e., Surging *Yang*), *daying* point (ST-5 who, i.e., Great Reception), *renying* point (ST-9 who, i.e., Man's Prognosis), *qichong* point (ST-30 who, i.e., *Qi* Thoroughfare), etc.

[2] The foot greater-*yang* bladder channel and foot lesser-*yang* gallbladder channel nearly have no pulsating points of vessels. However, the two channels become pulsating, large and rapid in this case: These two channels nearly have no pulsating points of vessels on them. In this condition, fury makes the *yang qi* disordered, so they become pulsating, large and rapid.

[3] Force the patient to starve: Eat little or nothing.

⁴ Foods enter the *yin* : Foods are transformed into the essential *qi* by the spleen. So we say that foods enter the *yin* .

⁵ So, if foods are deprived, the disease will terminate without the source of the *yang qi* : As if the fire-wood is pulled out from beneath the cauldron.

⁶ Take the Beverage of Raw Iron Powders, which can lower the *qi* swiftly : Raw iron powders are produced by hammering during smelting iron. They could be soaked by water, then the beverage could be taken to treat the disease. They pertain to metal, and are cold and heavy in nature. So, they are very good at lowering heat, tranquilizing the mind, untying binding, transforming phlegm, cooling the liver fire, and slaking fury.

Yang Carbuncle and *Yin* Carbuncle

5.19   Eighty-first Article

Yang *Carbuncle and* **Yin** *Carbuncle · The Divine Pivot* (*excerpt*)

5.19.1   Original article

The nutritive blood and defensive *qi* circle endlessly, corresponding to the upper heaven and lower earth. If cold evil dwells in the channels, the blood will be congealed. When the blood is congealed, obstruction appears. The obstruction causes the defensive *qi* to accumulate and fail to circle, so carbuncles occur. If the cold turns to be heat, the flesh will rot due to the heat, and pus will be produced by rotting. If the pus cannot be discharged, the tendons will decay. The decayed tendons will impair the bones. The impaired bones will cause the marrow to be reduced. The carbuncle is not at the joint, thus its heat cannot be discharged. The blood there becomes diminished and empty. The tendons, bones and flesh cannot be nourished. The channels are ruined and leaking. The heat steams the five *zang*-organs. The *zang*-organs are damaged, so death befalls.

Commentary

This article talks about the pathogen and pathomechanism of carbuncles. When the cold evil dwelling in the channels affects the running of the blood, local muscular striae appear to be red, swollen, hot and painful. So carbuncles form.

If carbuncles have formed, the flesh will putrefy and pus will be produced. Doctors should timely drain the pus, or it will result in decayed tendons, damaged bones, reduced marrow and desiccated blood. Finally, the channels will be ruined, and the heat will steam the five *zang*-organs resulting in death.

This article implies that the therapeutic methods, such as promoting blood circulation, transforming blood stasis, clearing heat, resolving toxin, incising to drain the pus, and tonifying to support the inside, are applicable.

5.19.2 Original article

The Emperor asked: "How can you differentiate a *yang* carbuncle from a *yin* carbuncle?"

Uncle Qi answered: "The nutritive *qi* lingers in the channels. Then the blood is congealed and stands still. When the blood stands still, obstruction of the defensive *qi* ensues. The obstruction then induces heat. The great heat does not terminate. The flesh decays due to the over-flourishing heat, and pus is produced due to the decaying of the flesh. However, the heat does not sink. The bones and marrow are not made withered, and the five *zang*-organs are not damaged. So it is called a *yang* carbuncle."

The Emperor asked: "What is a *yin* carbuncle?"

Uncle Qi answered: "The heat is overwhelming and sinks under the muscles and skin. The tendons and marrow are made withered. The five *zang*-organs are contaminated. The blood and *qi* are exhausted there. Under this carbuncle, all the tendons, bones and muscles are not intact. So it is called a *yin* carbuncle. The local skin of a *yin* carbuncle is darkish, gloomy and solid like the nape skin of an ox, whereas the local skin of a *yang* carbuncle is thin and glossy. These are its symptoms."

Commentary

This article discusses the differentiation between a *yang* carbuncle and a *yin* carbuncle. *Yang* carbuncle has *yang* symptoms, and is often seen as manifesting redness, swelling, heat, pain, thin and glossy skin, and a shallow location. Easy recovery after festering and pus-draining is also shown. A *yin* carbuncle has *yin* symptoms. It is often seen as having dark and gloomy skin color, broad swelling or flatness, no heat, a deep location, and thin pus after festering or cold and thick and foul pus. Difficulty in shrinkage of the sore, and a tendency to sink that may induce unfavorable changes are demonstrated as well.

5.20   Sixtieth Article

Jade Board · The Divine Pivot (*excerpt*)

Original article

The Emperor asked: "When the disease begins, immoderate joy and anger, improper diet, lack of the *yin qi*, surplus of the *yang qi*, and standstill of the nutritive *qi*, may induce a carbuncle. The *yin* and *yang* are impeded,[1] and two heats wrestle,[2] then pus is produced. Could little needles be used?"

Uncle Qi answered: "Sages usually expel the pus in a timely fashion because the evil cannot be allowed to stay there long. So, two conflicting troops confront face to face with flags fluttering, then white knives are spread over the battle field. This matter is not a day's scheme. Enabling its people to be strictly disciplined and its soldiers to survive the war is not a day's training or an instant's teaching that can be acquired. Until the body has been afflicted with carbuncle and purulent blood has gathered, the little needles are useless, aren't they? The generation of a carbuncle and formation of pus are not from the heaven or the earth, but due to gradual accumulation. So, the sages treat the carbuncle before its formation, whereas the stupid doctors treat it after the formation of the pus."

The Emperor asked: "When a carbuncle has formed and the pus has been produced, how does one treat the disease?"

Uncle Qi answered: "If pus has been produced, it will be ten deaths and one survival. Therefore, the sages make perfect prescriptions to prevent its formation. These prescriptions were recorded on the bamboo slips and silk to pass generation after generation without end so that nobody may suffer from pus formation and death."

The Emperor asked: "Since a carbuncle has formed and purulent blood has been produced, could we use little needles?"

Uncle Qi answered: "Treat big carbuncles with big needles. It is meritorious. Treat big carbuncles with little needles. It is pernicious. So, if a carbuncle has purulent blood, only the healing stone, sword needle and sharp-edged needle[3] should be selected."

The Emperor asked: "Couldn't the patients survive these pernicious conditions?[4]"

Uncle Qi answered: "The crucial point stands at the favorableness or unfavorableness (of the symptoms)."

The Emperor said: "Go on please with the favorableness and unfavorableness."

Uncle Qi continued: "Ulceration, blue color at the whites of the eyes, and shrunken colored parts of the eyes[5] are the first unfavorable condition. Vomiting after taking medicines[6] is the second unfavorable condition. Abdominal pain with great thirst[7] is the third unfavorable condition. Uncomfortable shoulders and neck[8] are the fourth unfavorable condition. Hoarse voice and lifeless color[9] are the fifth unfavorable condition. Except for these, all is favorable."

Commentary

These segments underscore the prevention, incipient diagnosis and early treatment of carbuncles. They also suggest five kinds of unfavorable exacerbated conditions. The evils sink. The five zang-organs are hurt. The stomach qi collapses. The fluids and blood are exhausted. These conditions are unfavorable, and forebode bad prognoses.

Annotation

[1] The yin and yang are impeded: The nutritive qi and defensive qi are impeded.

[2] Two heats wrestle: Exogenous heat and produced heat due to obstruction of the nutritive qi and defensive qi.

[3] Sword needle and sharp-edged needle: They are two kinds of the nine needles, which are used in acupuncture or operation. The sword needle is like a sword in shape, and it is often used to incise to expel pus or blood. The sharp-edged needle has three edges, so it is also called the three-edged needle, and it is often used to heal old intractable diseases.

[4] These pernicious conditions: Due to inappropriate treatments or worsening of the disease.

[5] Blue color at the whites of the eyes, and shrunken colored parts of the eyes: The lungs, liver and kidneys are all impaired.

[6] Vomiting after taking medicines: The stomach qi collapses.

[7] Abdominal pain with great thirst: Abdominal pain suggests that evils have entered the inside. Thirst reveals over-flourishing fire and impaired fluids.

[8] Uncomfortable shoulders and neck: The three hand yang channels pass along the shoulders; the three hand yang channels, the three foot yang channels, and the governing channel pass through the neck. Hence, the shoulders and neck become uncomfortable. It expresses that these

channels are all affected by evils.

⁹ Hoarse voice and lifeless color: Hoarse voice means exhausted lungs. Lifeless color suggests exhausted five *zang*-organs.

Chapter Six
Diagnostic Methods

Diagnostic methods are the means used to collect clinical data, which are analyzed with the theories of *yin-yang*, five elements, *zang*-organs and manifestations, channels and network-channels, pathogens and pathomechanisms, etc., so as to obtain references to syndrome identification and treatment determination. Hence, the applications of diagnostic methods are directly pertinent to syndrome identification and treatment determination.

The Medical Classic of the Yellow Emperor has many references to diagnostic methods. Some are discussed in special articles, and some are found in various chapters and articles. In the times when *The Medical Classic of the Yellow Emperor* was compiled, doctors underscored the importance of diagnostic methods. They had accumulated abundant experiences, and had gained brilliant achievements.

The diagnostic methods that people utilized from *The Medical Classic of the Yellow Emperor* encompass four points: observation, olfaction and auscultation, interrogation, and pulse-feeling and palpation. These were called the four examinations in later eras. Notwithstanding, some concrete methods in the four examinations are rarely used in praxis today due to causes of historical limitations, people always adhere to their ideological ways and theoretical viewpoints. The development of diagnostics in TCM has vastly benefited from these bases.

6.1   Eleventh Article

Discussion of Differentiations Among the Five Zang-Organs·
The Plain Questions (excerpt)

Original article

The Emperor asked: "Why is only the *qi*-opening pulse[1] dominated by the five *zang*-organs?"

Uncle Qi answered: "The stomach is the sea of water and grains, and the great source of the six *fu*-organs. The five flavors enter the mouth, and are stored in the stomach to nourish the *qi* of the five *zang*-organs. The *qi*-opening also pertains to the hand greater-*yin* lung channel.[2] So, the *qi* of the five *zang*-organs and six *fu*-organs all stems from the stomach, and is shown at the *qi*-opening with concentration. Thus, the five smells go into the nose and are stored in the heart and lungs. If the heart and lungs are unhealthy, the nose will not be smooth.

"In any treatment, a doctor should examine the neck and wrist pulses, feel the pulses, and observe the patient's spirit and thought and his disease. Do not discuss the supreme virtues[3] with those who are addicted to ghosts and gods. Do not remark upon the supreme techniques[4] with those who are abhorrent of needles and healing stones. Do not cure those who refuse treatment, or it is not meritorious."

Commentary

This section mainly states the basic principle that why exclusively taking the wrist pulse can determine diseases. Because the *qi*-opening belongs to the pulsating vessel of the hand greater-*yin* lung channel; the lungs govern the *qi* and face the hundred vessels. The lung channel starts from the middle-warmer's spleen and stomach, which are the great source of the essential *qi* of the five *zang*-organs and six *fu*-organs. So, the conditions of the *zang-fu* organs, channels, blood vessels, *qi* and blood can be revealed at the wrist pulse.

The article also mentions that doctors should not discuss the supreme virtues with those who are addicted to ghosts and gods. This idea sufficiently reflects the academic materialism of *The Medical Classic of the Yellow Emperor*.

Annotation

   [1] The *qi*-opening pulse: i.e., wrist pulse. It is also called the vessel-opening pulse, refer-
ring to a segment of the artery near the wrist, about three fingers long at the forearm. This segment
pertains to the pulsating vessel of the hand greater-*yin* lung channel. The lungs govern the *qi*.
Thus, the debilitation or exuberance of the *qi* is shown here, and it is called the *qi*-opening pulse.
The lungs face the hundred vessels, and the hundred vessels converge here, so it is also called the
vessel-opening pulse. The segment starts from the *taiyuan* point (LU-9 who, i.e., Great Abyss)
and is one point nine thumb-widths or thereabouts in length.

   [2] The *qi*-opening also pertains to the hand greater-*yin* lung channel: The *qi*-opening is the
pulsating vessel of the hand greater-*yin* lung channel.

   [3] The supreme virtues: Refer to medical theories.

   [4] The supreme techniques: Refer to skills of needles and healing stones.

6.2   Seventeenth Article

Discussion of Profundity and Subtlety of Pulse Essentials·
The Plain Questions (excerpt)

6.2.1   Original article

The Emperor asked: "What about pulse-feeling?"

Uncle Qi answered: "Ordinarily, pulse-feeling is taken at dawn when the *yin qi* has not moved, and the *yang qi* has not been dispersed.[1] Foods have not been taken. The channels have not been exuberant. The blood vessels are harmonious, and the *qi* and blood have not been disordered. So, abnormal pulses can be inspected.

"Feeling the movements or quietness of the pulse, a doctor should look at the spirit in the eyes,[2] and inspect the five colors of the complexion. The excess or shortage of the five *zang*-organs, strength or weakness of the six *fu*-organs, and exuberance or debilitation of the appearance should be observed. Consult all the information to predict death and life."

Commentary

This article points out that the proper time to take pulse is at dawn when the *qi* and blood are still tranquil without external disturbance and the pulse is the truest. Yet in clinical practice, it is impossible to serve any patient at dawn. So, the major premise of this article is that patients should keep calm and get rid of any external factors that may cause interference.

This article mentions the pulse-feeling, observing the eyes, inspecting the five colors, etc. These processes explain that pulse-taking should be combined with observation, olfaction and auscultation, and interrogation to meet the demand of correlation of the four examinations.

Annotation

[1] At dawn when the *yin qi* has not moved, and the *yang qi* has not been dispersed: There have not been works at dawn, so the *yin qi* has not moved and the *yang qi* has not been dispersed.

[2] Look at the spirit in the eyes: The spirit of the whole body can rush upward to the eyes.

6.2.2   Original article

The blood vessels are the house of the blood.[1] If the pulse is long,[2] the *qi* is normal. If the pulse is short, the *qi* is unhealthy. If the pulse is rapid, there is vexation. If the pulse is full, the disease is being exacerbated.[3] If the upper pulses of the body are exuberant, there are panting and fullness. If the lower pulses of the body are exuberant, there is abdominal distention.[4] If the pulse is regularly interrupted, it indicates feeble *qi*. If the pulse is thready, the *qi* is scant.[5] If the pulse is uneven, it is a painful heart.[6] If the pulse comes like a rushing spring, the disease is exasperated and the color becomes lifeless.[7] If the pulse leaves faintly like a broken string, it is fatal.[8]

The spirit in the eyes and the five colors seen in the complexion show how *qi* blooms. A healthy red complexion is like cinnabar wrapped in white silk,[9] while an unhealthy red complexion resembles hematite.[10] The healthy white complexion resembles goose feathers, while the unhealthy white complexion glistens like salt. The healthy blue complexion is evocative of the gloss of blue jade,[11] while the unhealthy blue complexion is flat like blue paint. The healthy yellow complexion resembles realgar wrapped in silk, while the unhealthy yellow complexion resembles yellow soil. The healthy black complexion is lustrous like heavy lacquer, while the unhealthy black complexion is like gloomy dark earth.

If the genuine colors of the five *zang*-organs are exposed,[12] the patient's life will not be long. The eyes are what look at all things, differentiate white from black, and check the short and the long. If the patient feels a long thing to be a short one or regards the white as black, this indicates that the essence has become weakened.

Commentary

This article makes color comparisons with concrete materials to enunciate vividly the healthy and unhealthy manifestations of the five colors. Distinguishing the five colors during observation yields significant information. If the color is iridescent, moist, translucent and not fully exhibited, it indicates the essential *qi* of the *zang-fu* organs is strong, and the prognosis is good. If the color is withered, murkily grey and flat, or the intense colors of the *zang*-organs are exhibited, it suggests the essential *qi* of the *zang*-organs is exhausted, and the prognosis is poor.

Observing the spirit in the eyes is also an important part of observation. Because all essential *qi* of the five *zang*-organs and six *fu*-organs flows upward to the eyes, changes in vision, especially the luster in the eyes, indicate the abundance or depletion of the essential *qi* of the five *zang*-organs. Ordinarily, spirited eyes and clear vision suggest that the essential *qi* is strong. Dispirited eyes and abnormal vision suggest that the essential *qi* is exhausted. Therefore, observing the eyes is significant in arriving at a diagnosis.

Annotation

[1] The blood vessels are the house of the blood: Blood runs in the blood vessels, so the blood vessels are the house of the blood, yet the blood is pushed forward by the *qi*.

[2] The pulse is long: It means that the body of pulse is long.

[3] If the pulse is rapid, there is vexation. If the pulse is full, the disease is being exacerbated: If the pulse pulsates more than five times during an inhalation and an exhalation, it is rapid. Rapid pulse suggests heat, so there is vexation. Full pulse reveals prevailing evils and a developing degree of seriousness.

[4] If the upper pulses of the body are exuberant, there are panting and fullness. If the lower pulses of the body are exuberant, there is abdominal distention: If the upper pulses of the body are exuberant, the evils congest at the upper part of the body, so there are panting and fullness. If the lower pulses of the body are exuberant, the evils linger at the lower part of the body, so there is abdominal distention.

[5] If the pulse is regularly interrupted, it indicates feeble *qi*. If the pulse is thready, the *qi* is scant: If the pulse is slow and weak with a regular interval, it reveals feeble *qi* of the *zang*-organs. The thready pulse means the pulse is as thin as a thread under the fingers. It dominates all deficiencies, impairment caused by work, deficient blood, and scanty *qi*.

[6] If the pulse is uneven, it is a painful heart: An uneven pulse suggests that the pulse is little uneven and not so smooth as a light knife scraping bamboo. It dominates deficient, scant *qi* and blood, or stagnant *qi* and blood stasis.

[7] If the pulse comes like a rushing spring, the disease is exasperated and the color becomes lifeless: If the pulse comes like a rushing spring, this suggests that the evils are prevailing and the disease is worsening. All colors stem from the blood, so the color becomes lifeless.

[8] If the pulse leaves faintly like a broken string, it is fatal: The pulse is so faint and weak that it is hardly perceptible. If the pulse leaves like a broken string, there will be death.

[9] Cinnabar wrapped in white silk: Dimly ruddy and not intensely exposed. Any color in the complexion that is iridescent, moist and translucent is healthy, while any hue that is flat, withered and exposed is unhealthy.

[10] Hematite: It seems reddish-brown, murkily grey without gloss.

[11] Blue jade: It seems blue, bright and moist with luster.

[12] The genuine colors of the five *zang*-organs are exposed: The essential *qi* of the five *zang*-organs transforms into the five colors. If the colors are fully exhibited on the surface, the essential *qi* has escaped storage, indicating the imminent collapse of the genuine *qi*, followed by death.

6.2.3 Original article

The five *zang*-organs keep the essential *qi* inside. The evil abounds in the middle-warmer, and the *zang*-organs become full. The patient (with vacuous *qi*) is frightened due to the prevailing evil. The voice seems to sound from a chamber. This is because the *qi* of the middle-warmer is clouded by damp.[1] Weak, low and intermittent speech is due to deprivation of the *qi*. Failure to keep clothing and covers on, and abusive remark without regard to his relatives, are due to deranged spirit.[2] The granary fails to store, because the gates were not strong enough to hold in the stored *qi*.[3] The water spring cannot be stopped, because the bladder fails to store. One whose body can maintain such restraint will live; one whose body fails in this regard will die.

The five *zang*-organs form the foundation of the body's vigor.[4] The head is the house of the essential *qi* and spirit. If the head droops and the eyes sink, the essential *qi* and spirit will be deprived. The back is the house of the chest.[5] If the back is curved and the shoulders droop, the heart and lungs will be ruined. The loins are the house of the kidneys. If shaking and turning are incapable, the kidneys will be ruined. The knees are the house of the tendons.[6] If the patient cannot bend or stretch, and he is curved and must lean on things to walk, the tendons will be ruined. The bones are the house of the marrow. If the patient cannot stand long and vibrates when walking, the bones will be ruined. One who increases vigor will live; one who loses vigor will die.

Commentary

These two segments explain the connection between the strength and weakness of the essential *qi* of the five *zang*-organs and that of the body form. One whose body can maintain such restraint will live; one whose body fails in this regard will die. One who increases vigor will live; one who loses vigor will die. These processes reveal the prognosis of a disease. All these processes can be detected not only visually, but also through smell and hearing, as well as inquiring about the patient's symptoms. This approach embodies the application of the correlation of four examinations.

Annotation

[1] The evil abounds in the middle-warmer, and the *zang*-organs become full. The patient (with

vacuous qi) is frightened due to the prevailing evil. The voice seems to sound from a chamber. This is because the qi of the middle-warmer is clouded by damp: A person's voice originates from the kidneys, exits from the lungs, and converges at the middle-warmer. The kidneys are damaged by fear, and damp in the middle-warmer can produce stagnation. Then the kidneys cannot communicate with the lungs, so the voice seems muffled as if it sounds from a chamber.

[2] Failure to keep clothing and covers on, and abusive remark without regard to his relatives, are due to deranged spirit: Stripping the clothes shamelessly and cursing even his relatives suggest a deranged spirit. The heart governs the spirit. If deranged, it means that the heart fails to restrain its essential qi.

[3] The granary fails to store, because the gates were not strong enough to hold in the stored qi: The granary refers to the stomach and intestines. The gates refer to anus, pylorus, etc. Endless diarrhea will occur.

[4] The five $zang$-organs form the foundation of the body's vigor: As the qi of the $zang$-organs is full, the body is strong.

[5] The back is the house of the chest: The heart and lungs stay in the chest, and their transport points are on the back, so the back is the house of the chest.

[6] The knees are the house of the tendons: The liver dominates the tendons. However, among all the tendons that link up with all joints to support the body, most of them exist around the knees and ankles.

6.2.4 Original article

The Emperor asked: "How does the pulse change with the four seasons? How can we know where the disease occurs? How do we recognize a disease's variations? How do we know the disease has suddenly arrived at the interior? Or the disease has suddenly come to the exterior? Could you explain these five matters?"

Uncle Qi answered: "The pulse variations correspond to the running of the heaven and earth. It is so vast and subtle! Outside everything and inside the six directions, every variation of the heaven and earth corresponds to that of the *yin* and *yang*. Spring's warmth becomes summer's heat, and the brisk of coolness of autumn becomes winter's piercing cold.

"The pulse changes with the seasonal changes. The spring pulse corresponds to a pair of compasses.[1] The summer pulse corresponds to a square.[2] The autumn pulse corresponds to the seam of a balance.[3] The winter pulse corresponds to a counterweight.[4]

"Therefore, during the forty-five days after the Winter Solstice,[5] the *yang qi* increases gradually while the *yin qi* decreases by degrees. During the forty-five days after the Summer Solstice,[6] the *yin qi* increases gradually while the *yang qi* decreases by degrees. The pulse variations are responsive to the changes of *yin* and *yang* of the four seasons. If they fail to be responsive, we will be able to foresee the death date according to the changes of pulse and seasons. The subtlety exists in the pulse. It is an inspection that can on no account be neglected.

"There is a principle of inspection that should be started from the *yin* and *yang*. There is a usual way of beginning that should be generated from the five elements. There is a law of generation that should be consulted with the four seasons.[7] We should not fail to supplement or drain appropriately, and should act in harmony with the heaven and earth. If we are acquainted with the law that man and nature are corresponding, life and death can be known. Hence, sounds correspond to the five musical scales. Colors correspond to the five elements. Pulses correspond to the *yin* and *yang*.

"Hence, when there is surplus *yin*, the patient dreams about fearfully wading through deep water.[8] When there is surplus *yang*, the patient dreams about a big fire, burning and scorching.[9] When the *yin* and *yang* are both at a surplus, the patient dreams about killing and casualties.[10] When the surplus is in the upper part of the body, flying dreams occur. When the surplus is in the lower part of the body, falling dreams occur.[11] When excessively sated, dreams of giving things to others occur. When excessively hungry, dreams of taking things from others occur.

"Overwhelming liver *qi* provokes angry dreams. Overwhelming lung *qi* provokes weeping in dreams.[12] When infested by short worms,[13] there are dreams about public congregation. When infested by long worms,[14] there are dreams about fighting and casualties.

"Therefore, pulse-taking has principles, yet modesty and calmness are most precious.[15] The pulse in spring is slightly floating as if fish swims in waves.[16] The pulse in summer is at the skin, so floating as if all things are abundant.[17] The pulse in autumn sinks underneath the skin as if dormant worms will burrow to hide.[18] The pulse in winter is near the bones as if worms hibernate and gentlemen hide in rooms.[19] Hence the saying: To know the *zang*-organs inside, doctors can press deeply to acquire the information. To know the channels outside, pulse-feeling enables the doctors to master clearly from the end to the beginning. These six items[20] are the great law of pulse-feeling."

Commentary

These segments elucidate the pulse's correspondence to the four seasons, based on the standpoint that man and nature correspond. During the regular natural changes, i.e., spring warmth, summer heat, autumn cool and winter cold, or spring generation, summer growth, autumn reaping and winter storage, the human pulse correspondingly reveals spring's compasses, summer's square, autumn's seam of balance, and winter's counter-weight. As a matter of fact, this phenomenon reveals the rhythm of the running *qi* and blood and their regular changes over the year. These four kinds of pulses are normal ones during the four seasons, not morbid ones. Being familiar with this can help us inspect pulse more accurately.

Dreams of men can also be divided into the *yin* and *yang*. They could be physiological or pathogenic. Interrogating about different dreams may assist us to learn the prosperity or decline of the *yin* and *yang* and *zang-fu* organs, so as to know the origin of a disease.

The article accentuates that "pulse-taking has principles, yet modesty and calmness are most precious." It has a two-sided meaning. On the one hand, doctors should be tranquil and focused to prevent distracting thoughts from interfering with the reading of complex pulses. On the other hand, patients should be calm and quiet so that real pulses are exhibited.

Annotation

[1] The spring pulse corresponds to a pair of compasses: A pair of compasses refers to round articles. The spring *qi* grows; it is round, lively and moving like a pair of compasses. The pulse corresponds to the spring *qi*, hence the pulse is round and slippery.

[2] The summer pulse corresponds to a square: A square refers to square objects. Square objects are square, upright and prosperous. So too is the summer pulse, which is surging, full, slippery and rapid.

[3] The autumn pulse corresponds to the seam of a balance: The autumn pulse feels like a feather floating on the surface of a pond. This pulse is light, uneven and dissipated like the style of the seam of a balance. We aim at its balance.

[4] The winter pulse corresponds to a counterweight: Winter dominates storage. The winter pulse sinks like a counterweight in a well, hiding in the depths.

[5] The Winter Solstice: Dec. 21, 22, or 23.

[6] The Summer Solstice: Jun. 21 or 22.

[7] There is a principle of inspection that should be started from the *yin* and *yang*. There is a usual way of beginning that should be generated from the five elements. There is a law of generation that should be consulted with the four seasons: These sentences suggest that we should keep in mind the *yin*, *yang*, five elements, and four seasons when feeling pulse.

[8] When there is surplus *yin*, the patient dreams about fearfully wading through deep water: Water is *yin*; fear is the emotion associated with the water element. So these factors are revealed through the motif of being in dangerously deep water.

[9] When there is surplus *yang*, the patient dreams about a big fire, burning and scorching: Fire is *yang*, prompting the imaginary of flames and burning.

[10] When the *yin* and *yang* are both at a surplus, the patient dreams about killing and casualties: With both *yin* and *yang* excess, water and fire attack one another. Their contention evokes dreams of killing and casualties.

[11] When the surplus is in the upper part of the body, flying dreams occur. When the surplus is in the lower part of the body, falling dreams occur: With a surplus in the upper part of the body, the *qi* tends to rise. The liver, storing the *yang* soul with ascendant *qi*, follows this rising motion and produces the flying dreams. With a surplus in the lower part of the body, the *qi* tends to descend. The lungs, housing the *yin* soul with its descending *qi*, follows this motion and produces falling dreams. These occurrences also illustrate the quality of the two corresponding elements: wood (the liver) floats and metal (the lungs) sinks.

[12] Overwhelming liver *qi* provokes angry dreams. Overwhelming lung *qi* provokes weeping in dreams: The surplus liver *qi* ascends, and anger is the emotion associated with the liver, so the liver reveals its surplus *qi* through anger in dreams. The surplus lung *qi* descends, and grief is the emotion associated with the lungs, so the lung *qi* reveals its surplus through weeping in dreams.

[13] Short worms: Pinworms.

[14] Long worms: Roundworms.

[15] Yet modesty and calmness are most precious: Doctors should keep calm and modest so that the true pulse can be detected with concentration.

[16] The pulse in spring is slightly floating as if fish swims in waves: The pulse receives the spring *qi*, then it is slightly floating but not exposed utterly. So it seems as if fish swims in waves.

[17] The pulse in summer is at the skin, so floating as if all things are abundant: The pulse in summer is floating, full and prosperous at the skin like all things are abundant enough.

[18] The pulse in autumn sinks underneath the skin as if dormant worms will burrow to hide: In autumn, the *yang qi* begins to decline. The pulse sinks under the skin like dormant worms burrow to conceal themselves.

[19] The pulse in winter is near the bones as if worms hibernate and gentlemen hide in rooms: In winter, the *yang qi* is stored inside, so the pulse sinks to the bones like hibernating worms and gentlemen enclosed in rooms.

[20] These six items: Refer to the spring, summer, autumn, winter, interior and exterior mentioned in this article.

6.2.5 Original article

（We ordinarily divide the cubital skin into three parts.）[1] As to the proximal part, the ulnar side serves the soft ribs,[2] the radial side serves the kidneys, and the middle area serves the abdomen. As to the middle part, the radial side of the left arm serves the liver, and its ulnar side serves the diaphragm; the radial side of the right arm serves the stomach, and its ulnar side serves the spleen. As to the distal part, the radial side of the right arm serves the lungs, and its ulnar side serves the chest; the radial side of the left arm serves the heart, and its ulnar side serves the breast.

The inner surface of the forearm serves the front of the body, and the outer surface of the forearm serves the back of the body. The distal end of the cubital skin serves the chest and throat, and the proximal end of the cubital skin serves the lower abdomen, waist, hips, knees, shanks and feet.

Commentary

This article mentions the inspection of the cubital skin, which is rarely used today. It is an archaic diagnostic method. Special areas of the cubital skin correspond to the *zang*-organs, *fu*-organs, and other organs. Doctors can tell the cold or heat property of a disease, and also the waning or waxing of the fluids, by inspecting the cold, heat, smoothness or unevenness of the cubital skin. Nowadays, it is worth application in some diseases or syndromes, especially febrile diseases.

Annotation

[1] We ordinarily divide the cubital skin into three parts: The cubital skin here refers to the inner surface of the forearm from the wrist to elbow. It is divided into three parts, which are respectively called distal part, middle part and proximal part.

[2] The soft ribs: Equivalent to the cartilage of the 11th and 12th ribs.

6.3   Eighteenth Article

Discussion of Manifestations of Pulse Qi of
Healthy People · The Plain Questions

6.3.1   Original article

The Emperor asked: "What about the pulse of healthy people?"

Uncle Qi answered: "A man exhales once while the pulse beats twice, and he inhales once while the pulse beats twice, and then the pulse beats once again in the interval. This man is called a healthy person who has no ailments. We often measure the patient's pulse in contrast to our own. If the doctor is healthy, he can tranquilize his own breath to measure the patient's pulse.

"If one exhales once while the pulse beats once, and inhales once while the pulse beats once, it is called scant *qi*.[1] One exhales once while the pulse beats three times, and inhales once while the pulse beats three times agitatedly; if the cubital skin is hot, the patient suffers from a febrile disease;[2] if the cubital skin is not hot and the pulse is slippery, the patient is afflicted with wind;[3] if the pulse is uneven, there is an impediment disease.[4] If one exhales once, yet the pulse beats more than four times, it is fatal. If the pulse disappears and fails to come again, it is fatal. If the pulse is abruptly slow and suddenly rapid, it is deadly as well.[5]"

Commentary

This article introduces the basic methods of tranquilizing breath to inspect pulse and of discriminating normal pulse from abnormal pulse or fatal pulse. These methods are still used today. Moreover, the article also introduces the method of correlating cubital skin inspection with pulse-taking to determine febrile disease, wind disease, and impediment disease. The correlation of cubital skin inspection and pulse-taking is valuable to some degree in clinical practice.

Annotation

[1] If one exhales once while the pulse beats once, and inhales once while the pulse beats once, it is called scant *qi*: The blood vessels are the tunnels for the blood flow, which is propelled by the *qi*. When the patient's pulse is only a half in contrast to healthy people. It suggests that the right

qi is exhausted, so it is called scant *qi*.

[2] If the cubital skin is hot, the patient suffers from a febrile disease: If the cubital skin is hot, the patient's whole body must be hot. When the pulse is agitatedly rapid and the body is hot, the patient must suffer a febrile disease.

[3] If the cubital skin is not hot and the pulse is slippery, the patient is afflicted with wind: The pulse is slippery and the cubital skin is not hot. It indicates overwhelming *yang* evils. So the patient should be afflicted with wind. However, when the wind harms men, it is variable and does not only stay at the skin, so the cubital pulse is not hot.

[4] If the pulse is uneven, there is an impediment disease: The unevenness of the blood indicates dissonant blood, so the patient should be afflicted with an impediment disease.

[5] If one exhales once, yet the pulse beats more than four times, it is fatal. If the pulse disappears and fails to come again, it is fatal. If the pulse is abruptly slow and suddenly rapid, it is deadly as well: Four beats in an exhalation are too excessive and mean the essence is deprived. The pulse disappearing and failing to come again indicates that the original *qi* is exhausted. An abruptly slow and suddenly rapid pulse indicates a collapse of the *yin* and *yang*.

6.3.2   Original article

"The pulse *qi* of healthy people is endowed with the stomach *qi*. The stomach *qi* is the normal pulse *qi* of healthy people.[1] If one's pulse has no stomach *qi*, it is unfavorable, and the patient will perish.

"The normal spring pulse is slightly string-like with stomach *qi*.[2] If the pulse is excessively string-like with scant stomach *qi*, the liver suffers. If only string-like without stomach *qi*, it is fatal.[3] If floating pulse is also seen with stomach *qi*, the disease will occur in the autumn. If extremely floating, the disease will occur immediately.[4] All genuine *qi* of the *zang*-organs spreads in the liver, and the liver stores the *qi* of the tendons and membranes.[5]

"The normal summer pulse is slightly surging and full with stomach *qi*.[6] If the pulse is excessively surging and full with scant stomach *qi*, the heart suffers. If only surging and full without stomach *qi*, it is fatal. If sinking pulse is also seen with stomach *qi*, the disease will occur in the winter. If extremely sinking, the disease will occur at once. All genuine *qi* of the *zang*-organs flows to the heart, and the heart stores the *qi* of the blood and vessels. The normal pulse of late summer is slightly soft and weak with stomach *qi*. If the pulse is excessively weak with scant stomach *qi*, the spleen suffers. If excessively weak and not accompanied by stomach *qi*, it is fatal. If sinking pulse is seen with the soft and weak pulse, the disease will occur in the winter. If extremely sinking, the disease will occur immediately.[7] All genuine *qi* of the *zang*-organs moistens the spleen, and the spleen stores the *qi* of the flesh.

"The normal autumn pulse is slightly floating with stomach *qi*.[8] If the pulse is excessively floating with scant stomach *qi*, the lungs suffer. If only floating without stomach *qi*, it is fatal. If string-like pulse accompanies floating pulse, the disease will occur in the spring. If extremely string-like, the disease will occur at once.[9] The genuine *qi* of the *zang*-organs is as high as the lungs, and the lungs move the nutritive blood, defensive *qi*, *yin* and *yang*.

"The normal winter pulse is slightly sinking with stomach *qi*.[10] If the pulse is excessively sinking with scant stomach *qi*, the kidneys suffer. If only sinking without stomach qi, it is fatal. If surging and full pulse accompanies sinking pulse, the disease will occur in the summer. If extremely surging and full, the disease will occur at once.[11] All genuine qi of the *zang*-organs descends to the kidneys, and the kidneys store the qi of the bones and marrow.

"The big network-channel of the stomach channel is called vacuous interior.[12] It penetrates the diaphragm, joins with the lungs, and exits from beneath the left breast. Its pulsation is palpable. The ancestral qi can be detected at this location. If the pulsations are frantic like panting, or beat rapidly with interruptions, the disease is in the middle-warmer.[13] If the pulsations beat irregularly with interruptions and remain replete and forceful under the fingers, there are accumulations in the stomach. If the pulsations disappear and do not come again, it is fatal.[14] If the pulsations can be seen through clothing, the ancestral qi leaks.[15]"

Commentary

These segments point out the significance that the pulse puts the stomach qi as its basis. They also introduce the normal pulses, abnormal pulses, and fatal pulses in the four seasons, and the diagnostic method of the vacuous interior.

In the spring and summer, the abnormal pulses are those that pertain to their curbing seasons; in the late summer, autumn and winter, the abnormal pulses are those that pertain to their curbed seasons. This condition demonstrates the complexity of pulse changes over the four seasons, yet they never exceed the relationship of overcontrolling or insulting among the five elements. The existence or non-existence and the amount of the stomach qi are crucial in perceiving the difference between normal and abnormal pulses, and recognizing the fatal pulses. When the stomach qi is scant, diseases occur; when it vanishes, death comes. The theory that the pulse puts the stomach qi as its basis had a far-reaching influence upon the development of pulse diagnosis in later eras. Perhaps, the theory of "stomach qi, spirit, and root" of the pulse stems from this idea.

Detecting the pulsation of the vacuous interior to measure the abundance or scarcity of the ancestral qi, could help us to determine the seriousness of a disease and whether death is imminent.

Annotation

[1] The stomach qi is the normal pulse qi of healthy people: The stomach is the acquired basis, and the origin of the qi. If the stomach qi shows at the pulse, we say that the pulse has stomach qi. Any pulse that is natural, graceful and unhurried is a pulse with stomach qi.

[2] The normal spring pulse is slightly string-like with stomach qi: The string-like pulse seems

long and like touching on a string.

³ If the pulse is excessively string-like with scant stomach *qi*, the liver suffers. If only string-like without stomach *qi*, it is fatal: An excessively string-like pulse with stomach *qi* indicates that the liver wood is overwhelming and losing its harmony, yet the stomach *qi* still exists, so the liver is ill. If the stomach *qi* vanishes, it is fatal.

⁴ If floating pulse is also seen with stomach *qi*, the disease will occur in the autumn. If extremely floating, the disease will occur immediately: The floating pulse is the normal pulse in autumn, yet it appears in the spring. This is an evil. However, the stomach *qi* still exists, so the disease will occur in the autumn. If the pulse is extremely floating, wood is overcontrolled by metal. It is not necessary to await the autumn's arrival, the disease will occur immediately.

⁵ All genuine *qi* of the *zang*-organs spreads in the liver, and the liver stores the *qi* of the tendons and membranes: In spring, the liver is on duty, so all genuine *qi* of the *zang*-organs spreads in the liver, which dominates the tendons and membranes.

⁶ The normal summer pulse is slightly surging and full with stomach *qi*: The surging and full pulse is also known as hook-like pulse. It comes prosperously and leaves weakly, evoking the shape of a hook.

⁷ If sinking pulse is seen with the soft and weak pulse, the disease will occur in the winter. If extremely sinking, the disease will occur immediately: The sinking pulse is the normal pulse in winter and pertains to water. The *yang qi* in late summer is very prosperous, yet the winter pulse appears. It shows that the fire-soil is so weak that the water overcontrols it. If the stomach *qi* still exists, the disease will occur in the winter. If the stomach *qi* vanishes, the disease will occur at once.

⁸ The normal autumn pulse is slightly floating with stomach *qi*: The floating pulse seems so light, vacuous and floating like touching a feather. Thus, the floating pulse here is also called feather-like pulse.

⁹ If string-like pulse accompanies floating pulse, the disease will occur in the spring. If extremely string-like, the disease will occur at once: The autumn sees a spring pulse. It shows that metal *qi* is so weak that wood insults it. If the stomach *qi* still exists, the disease will occur in the spring. If the stomach *qi* does not exist, the metal *qi* is so feeble that the disease will occur at once.

¹⁰ The normal winter pulse is slightly sinking with stomach *qi*: The sinking pulse is a deep pulse. Here, the sinking pulse is also called stone-like pulse.

¹¹ If surging and full pulse accompanies sinking pulse, the disease will occur in the summer. If extremely surging and full, the disease will occur at once: The winter sees a summer pulse. It shows that water is so weak that fire insults it.

¹² Vacuous interior: Where the apex of the heart pulsates, under the left breast at the fifth intercostal space.

¹³ If the pulsations are frantic like panting, or beat rapidly with interruptions, the disease is in the middle-warmer: It shows the *qi* of the middle-warmer fails to restrain the ancestral *qi*, so the disease is at the middle-warmer.

¹⁴ If the pulsations disappear and do not come again, it is fatal: The ancestral *qi* vanishes.

¹⁵ If the pulsations can be seen through clothing, the ancestral *qi* leaks: The ancestral *qi* should be stored and not be visibly spent. When seen through clothing, it means that the ancestral *qi* is leaking out.

6.3.3 Original article

"The excess or deficiency of the wrist pulse can be detected. If the wrist pulse feels short, headache occurs; if the wrist pulse feels long, there are pains of the feet and shins.[1] If the wrist pulse beats rapidly upward, there are pains of the shoulders and back.[2] If the wrist pulse feels sinking and solid, the disease occurs at the interior; if it feels floating and excessive, the disease occurs at the exterior.[3]

"If the wrist pulse feels deep, replete and forceful, there are accumulations at the rib-sides, and pains in the abdomen due to the accumulations.[4] If the wrist pulse feels sinking and rapid, chill and fever will occur.[5] If the wrist pulse feels excessive, slippery and solid, the disease occurs at the exterior; if it is small, replete and solid, the disease occurs at the interior.[6] If the wrist pulse feels small, weak and uneven, the disease will be a prolonged one; if it is slippery, floating and swift, the condition is new.[7]

"If the pulse feels string-like and tense, there may be hernia, conglomeration, and pain in the lower abdomen.[8] If the wrist pulse feels slippery, there may be a wind disease.[9] If the wrist pulse feels uneven, an impediment disease exists.[10] If the wrist pulse is slow and slippery, there is heat in the middle-warmer. If the wrist pulse is excessive and tense, abdominal distention will occur.[11]

"If the pulse is in accordance with the *yin* and *yang*, the disease will be easy to cure. If the pulse is not in accordance with the *yin* and *yang*, the disease will be difficult to cure.[12] If the pulse corresponds to the four seasons, nothing will be serious.[13] If the pulse does not correspond to the four seasons, or the disease is passed on from a *zang*-organ to its curbed *zang*-organ,[14] the disease will be hard to cure.

"If many blue vessels are visible in the arms, it is an indication of a loss of blood.[15] If the cubital skin is slack and the pulse is uneven, the patient will be slothful and somnolent.[16] If the cubital skin is hot and the pulse is excessive, it is an indication of a sudden loss of blood.[17] If the cubital skin is not smooth and the pulse is slippery, there will be profuse sweating.[18] If the cubital skin is cold and the pulse is thready, there will be diarrhea.[19] If the pulse is thick and the cubital skin is always hot, there is heat in the middle-warmer.[20]

"The patient with liver disease will die on the S7 and S8 days. The patient with heart disease will die on the S9 and S10 days. The patient suffering spleen disease will die on the S1 and S2 days. The patient suffering lung disease will die on the S3 and S4 days. The patient with kidney disease will die on the S5 and S6 days.

"Anyone will die when the genuine pulses of the *zang*-organs are exhibited.[21]

"If the neck pulse stirs and there are rapid panting and coughing, it is due to water imbalance.[22] If the eyelids swell slightly like a just awakened silkworm getting up, it is due to water imbalance.[23] If the urine is yellow and reddish and the patient has somnolence, there is jaundice.[24] If hungry even after having eaten, it is due to heat in the stomach.[25] If the face swells, it is due to wind.[26] If the feet and shins swell, it is due to water imbalance.[27] If the eyes are yellow, there is jaundice. If the hand lesser-*yin* pulse[28] of a woman stirs excessively, it is an indication of pregnancy.

"When the pulses are not attuned to the four seasons, they do not correspond to the normal shapes of the corresponding *zang*-organs.

"If the pulse is sinking and thready in spring and summer, while it is floating and large in autumn and winter, it is called discordance to the four seasons. If there is wind-heat, yet the pulse is quiet; if there are diarrhea and blood loss, yet the pulse is replete; if the disease occurs at the interior, yet the pulse is deficient; if the disease occurs at the exterior, yet the pulse is uneven and solid;[29] these conditions are all difficult to treat, and they are called contradiction to the four seasons."

Commentary

These segments mainly introduce the changes of the wrist pulse, their associated diseases, and the method of the correlation of wrist pulse and cubital skin. Through detecting variations of the wrist pulse, we can determine whether the disease occurs at the upper part, lower part, interior, or exterior. The slightness, seriousness, newness, or prolongation of a disease, and the wind, cold, or heat of a disease's attribute can be known. The impediment, pain, or distention about the major dominated disease, and the favorableness, unfavorableness, and prognoses of diseases could be mastered. Just as we say: The *qi*-opening is about two thumb-widths long; this is where death and life are determined.

Annotation

[1] If the wrist pulse feels short, headache occurs; if the wrist pulse feels long, there are pains of the feet and shins: The beat of the wrist pulse is felt under the fingers. When the *qi* of the wrist pulse is short, the *qi* must be deficient and fails to flow to the upper part of the body. As a result headache occurs, which suggests that the right *qi* is deficient in the upper part of the body. When the *qi* of the wrist pulse is long, the *qi* must be too exuberant and excessive in the lower part of the body. So pains occur in the feet and shins, suggesting that evils are prevailing in the lower part of the body.

[2] If the wrist pulse beats rapidly upward, there are pains of the shoulders and back: Beating rapidly upward to the touch of the fingers means the pulse is surging, large and rapid. This is the sign that the *yang* is exuberant and the fire is intense. The back is the *yang* of the body. When the *yang* fire is excessive, the shoulders and back will be painful.

[3] If the wrist pulse feels sinking and solid, the disease occurs at the interior; if it feels floating and excessive, the disease occurs at the exterior: The sinking pulse dominates the interior, and being solid means that *yang* is abundant. The floating pulse dominates the exterior, and the excessive one means the *yang* is strong.

[4] If the wrist pulse feels deep, replete and forceful, there are accumulations at the rib-sides, and pains in the abdomen due to the accumulations: The sinking pulse dominates the interior. A replete and forceful pulse suggests that accumulations do exist. So there are pains of the rib-sides and abdomen due to the accumulations.

[5] If the wrist pulse is sinking and rapid, chill and fever will occur: The sinking and rapid pulse indicates that heat exists inside. So chill and fever will occur due to this heat. That is to say, all lock-jaw and shudder are ascribed to the fire.

[6] If the wrist pulse feels excessive, slippery and solid, the disease occurs at the exterior; if it is small, replete and solid, the disease occurs at the interior: The excessive and slippery pulse pertains to *yang*. The small and replete pulse pertains to *yin*. The ill *yin* determines the disease to occur at the interior, whereas the ill *yang* determines the disease to occur at the exterior.

[7] If the wrist pulse feels small, weak and uneven, the disease will be a prolonged one; if it is slippery, floating and swift, the condition is new: The small and weak pulse signifies *qi* deficiency, and the uneven one signifies a shortage of blood. So the disease will be a prolonged one. The floating and slippery pulse is a *yang* one. The swift *yang* pulse indicates that evils are overwhelming. So the overwhelming evils and the developing tendency may cause a new disease.

[8] If the pulse feels string-like and tense, there may be hernia, conglomeration, and pain in the lower abdomen: The string-like and tense pulse suggests prevailing *yin* evils. So hernia, conglomeration, and pain in the lower abdomen will appear.

[9] If the wrist pulse feels slippery, there may be a wind disease: The wind is a *yang* evil, and it is mobile and variable. So the pulse is slippery.

[10] If the wrist pulse feels uneven, an impediment disease exists: The uneven pulse reveals coagulation of the blood and *qi*. So there is an impediment disease.

[11] If the wrist pulse is slow and slippery, there is heat in the middle-warmer. If the wrist pule

is excessive and tense, abdominal distention will occur: The slow pulse indicates that the spleen pulse is excessive, and the slippery one indicates the stomach fire is excessively exuberant. So, there is heat in the middle-warmer. The tense pulse indicates overwhelming cold evil, and the cold is replete inside. So the abdomen becomes full.

[12] If the pulse is in accordance with the *yin* and *yang*, the disease will be easy to cure. If the pulse is not in accordance with the *yin* and *yang*, the disease will be difficult to cure: A *yin* disease showing a *yin* pulse or a *yang* disease showing a *yang* pulse is in accord. A *yin* disease showing a *yang* pulse or a *yang* disease showing a *yin* pulse is not in accord.

[13] If the pulse corresponds to the four seasons, nothing will be serious: Namely, string-like pulse in spring, surging and full pulse in summer, floating pulse in autumn, and sinking pulse in winter.

[14] The disease is passed on from a *zang*-organ to its curbed *zang*-organ: e.g., the liver disease is passed onto the spleen; the spleen disease is passed onto the kidneys.

[15] If many blue vessels are visible in the arms, it is an indication of a loss of blood: If the channels have sufficient blood, the vessels will be red. If the channels lose their blood, blue vessels will be visible in the arms.

[16] If the cubital skin is slack and the pulse is uneven, the patient will be slothful and somnolent: The uneven pulse indicates insufficient blood. So the patient has slothfulness and somnolence.

[17] If the cubital skin is hot and the pulse is excessive, it is an indication of a sudden loss of blood: The excessive pulse indicates exuberant fire. The fire is so effulgent that it forces the blood to flow wildly. So a sudden loss of blood occurs.

[18] If the cubital skin is not smooth and the pulse is slippery, there will be profuse sweating: The uneven cubital skin indicates scant nutritive blood, and the slippery pulse indicates exuberant *yin* fire. So the deficient *yin* and exuberant *yang* lead to profuse sweating.

[19] If the cubital skin is cold and the pulse is thready, there will be diarrhea: The cold cubital skin suggests a deficiency of the spleen *yang*, because the spleen governs the muscles. The thready pulse exhibits a deficiency of the kidney *yang*. So the vacuous cold of the spleen and kidneys can cause diarrhea.

[20] If the pulse is thick and the cubital skin is always hot, there is heat in the middle-warmer: The thick pulse and always hot cubital skin suggest that the *yang qi* is in surplus. So there is heat in the middle-warmer.

[21] Anyone will die when the genuine pulses of the *zang*-organs are exhibited: If the genuine pulses of the *zang*-organs are exposed, when the curbing date comes, the patient will die at that time.

[22] If the neck pulse stirs and there are rapid panting and coughing, it is due to water imbalance: The neck pulse is namely the *renying* (ST-9 who, i.e., Man's Prognosis) pulse, which pertains to the foot bright-*yang* stomach channel. The water *qi* adversely flows upwards to attack the bright-*yang* stomach channel. So the neck pulse stirs. The water floods the lungs, and rapid panting and coughing occur.

[23] If the eyelids swell slightly like a just awakened silkworm getting up, it is due to water imbalance: The eyelids are where the stomach channel passes, and are dominated by the spleen. When water overflows the spleen and stomach, the eyelids swell slightly as if a silkworm just woke

up.

[24] If the urine is yellow and reddish and the patient has somnolence, there is jaundice: Usually, the damp-heat or cold-damp obstructs in the middle-warmer, so that the bile fails to flow in its normal way. So jaundice occurs, characterized by a yellow body, yellow eyes, and yellow urine. When the damp-heat rushes downward, the urine becomes yellow and reddish. The damp encumbers the flesh. So the patient has somnolence.

[25] If hungry even after having eaten, it is due to heat in the stomach: If the stomach is hot, digestion is quick and hunger easily recurs.

[26] If the face swells, it is due to wind: The *qi* of the six *yang* channels all converges at the face. When the wind assaults a man, the face is afflicted first. So face swelling is due to wind.

[27] If the feet and shins swell, it is due to water imbalance: The spleen and stomach govern the damp, and the kidneys and the bladder dispose of water. Their channels all run through the feet and shins. So swollen feet and shins are due to water imbalance.

[28] The hand lesser-*yin* pulse: Here, refers to the *shenmen* point (HT-7 who, i.e., Spirit Gate), which is on the transverse crease of the wrist, at the inner face of the arm.

[29] If there is wind-heat, yet the pulse is quiet; if there are diarrhea and blood loss, yet the pulse is replete; if the disease occurs at the interior, yet the pulse is deficient; if the disease occurs at the exterior, yet the pulse is uneven and solid: If there is wind-heat, the pulse should be floating and large, yet the pulse is sinking and quiet in this case. If a *yang* disease shows a *yin* pulse, it is morbid. If there are diarrhea and blood loss, the pulse should be sinking and thready; however, the pulse is replete and large in this case, revealing a *yin* disease with a *yang* pulse.

When a disease occurs at the interior, if the pulse is forceful, the *qi* of the middle-warmer must be exuberant. Then the disease will be easy to recover. However, the pulse is deficient in this case, so the disease will be difficult to treat. When the disease occurs at the exterior, if the pulse is floating and vacuous, the exterior disease will be easy to recover. However, the pulse is uneven and solid in this case, so the disease will be hard to treat.

6.3.4   Original article

"Men take water and grains as the basis of the sustenance, so men will die without them. If the pulse does not have the stomach *qi*, the patient will die as well. A pulse that is absent of the stomach *qi* means the genuine pulse of a *zang*-organ appears without the stomach *qi*. The pulse that is absent of the stomach *qi* can be detected. For example, the liver pulse is not string-like; the kidney pulse is not sinking.

"When the greater-*yang* pulse appears, it is surging, large and long.[1] When the lesser-*yang* pulse appears, it is suddenly rapid and abruptly slow, and suddenly short and abruptly long.[2] When the bright-*yang* pulse appears, it is floating, large and short.[3]"

Commentary

This article introduces the normal pulses in the six months. *The Medical Classic on Eighty-One Difficult Questions* adds, "When the greater-*yin* pulse appears, it is tight, large and long. When the lesser-*yin* pulse appears, it is tight, thready and slight. When the cold-*yin* pulse appears, it is sinking, short and substantial."

Annotation

[1] When the greater-*yang* pulse appears, it is surging, large and long: The greater-*yang* dominates June and July when the *yang qi* is most exuberant. So the pulse is surging, large and long.

[2] When the lesser-*yang* pulse appears, it is suddenly rapid and abruptly slow, and suddenly short and abruptly long: The lesser-*yang* dominates February and March when the *yang qi* is still faint and the *yin qi* still exists. So, the pulse with the *yin* and *yang* is concomitantly seen, and it is suddenly rapid and abruptly slow, and suddenly short and abruptly long.

[3] When the bright-*yang* pulse appears, it is floating, large and short: The bright-*yang* dominates April and May when the *yang qi* is not exuberant while the *yin qi* still exists. Although the pulse is floating and large, short sign is also exhibited. The floating and large pulse is *yang* and the short pulse is *yin*.

6.3.5   Original article

"When the pulse of the normal heart appears, it is as soft and sleek as touching a strand of pearls or pearl-like jades. This is the normal heart pulse.[1] The summer pulse takes the stomach *qi* as its basis.[2] When the pulse of the diseased heart comes, it is as rapid as panting and slightly curved. This is the diseased heart pulse.[3] When the pulse of the dying heart comes, it is curved like hooks. This is the fatal heart pulse.[4]

"When the pulse of the normal lungs appears, it is as gentle as dropping elm seeds. This is the normal lung pulse.[5] The autumn pulse takes the stomach *qi* as its basis. When the pulse of the diseased lungs comes, it is neither up nor down but is like touching hen feather. This is the diseased lung pulse.[6] When the pulse of the dying lungs comes, it feels like floating things and feathers blown in a wind. This is the fatal lung pulse.[7]

"When the pulse of the normal liver appears, it is as soft and weak as the end of a held long pole. This is the normal liver pulse.[8] The spring pulse takes the stomach *qi* as its basis. When the pulse of the diseased liver comes, it is full, replete and slippery like touching a long pole. This is the diseased liver pulse.[9] When the pulse of the dying liver comes, it is as taut as touching the string of a drawn bow. This is the fatal liver pulse.[10]

"When the pulse of the normal spleen appears, it is soft and natural as if a chicken walks in the field. This is the normal spleen pulse.[11] The late summer puts the stomach *qi* as its basis. When the pulse of the diseased spleen comes, it is replete, full and rapid like a hen lifting its feet. This is the diseased spleen pulse.[12] When the pulse of the dying spleen comes, it is sharp and hard like the beak of a crow or the claws of a bird, or it seems like the leakage of a roof or the flow of water. This is the fatal spleen pulse.[13]

"When the pulse of the normal kidneys appears, it is coherent, slippery, and slightly surging and full, and it is hard when touched. This is the normal kidney pulse.[14] The winter pulse puts the stomach *qi* as its basis. When the pulse of the diseased kidneys comes, it is as tight as a drawn vine and becomes harder when pressed. This is the diseased kidney pulse.[15] When the pulse of the dying kidneys comes, it is as taut as touching a fiercely tugged rope, or solid as if the fingers are flicking at a stone. This is the fatal kidney pulse.[16]"

Commentary

This article vividly depicts the normal pulses, the diseased pulses, and the fatal pulses of the five *zang*-organs (i.e., the five seasons). The article underlines that any pulse that is harmonious, graceful and smooth has stomach *qi*. Therefore, the main points to distinguish between the normal pulses and the ill or fatal pulses remain the exuberance or the decline, and the existence or the non-existence of the stomach *qi*. The stomach *qi* is extremely vital to a normal pulse.

Annotation

[1] When the pulse of the normal heart appears, it is as soft and sleek as touching a strand of pearls or pearl-like jades. This is the normal heart pulse: Touching a strand of pearls or pearl-like jades suggests that the pulse is excessive, full and sleek, namely, slightly surging and full which is the normal pulse of the heart (summer).

[2] The summer pulse takes the stomach *qi* as its basis: The heart pulse prevailsing in summer. It should have harmonious stomach *qi*, and the stomach *qi* should not be excessive.

[3] When the pulse of the diseased heart comes, it is as rapid as panting and slightly curved. This is the diseased heart pulse: It is as rapid as panting and slightly curved; the pulse is not so slippery as touching pearls. It fails to have harmonious stomach *qi*, so the heart becomes ill.

[4] When the pulse of the dying heart comes, it is curved like hooks. This is the fatal heart pulse: The pulse is only surging and full without the stomach *qi*. So this is called the fatal heart pulse.

[5] When the pulse of the normal lungs appears, it is as gentle as dropping elm seeds. This is the normal lung pulse: Dropping elm seeds suggest that the pulse is light, floating and gentle, namely, slightly floating that is the normal pulse of the lungs (autumn).

[6] When the pulse of the diseased lungs comes, it is neither up nor down but is like touching hen feather. This is the diseased lung pulse: Being neither up nor down means the pulse is uneven. Touching hen feather indicates that the pulse is lighter and more vacuous than elm seeds. So the lungs are unhealthy.

[7] When the pulse of the dying lungs comes, it feels like floating things and feathers blown in a wind. This is the fatal lung pulse: Floating things indicate vacuity and absence of root. Feathers blown in a wind mean mess and disorder. So, the pulse is only floating without stomach *qi*. This is the fatal lung pulse.

[8] When the pulse of the normal liver appears, it is as soft and weak as the end of a held long pole. This is the normal liver pulse: The end of a held long pole must be soft, that is to say, the pulse feels soft, string-like, and long. This is the normal pulse of the liver (spring).

[9] When the pulse of the diseased liver comes, it is full, replete and slippery like touching a long pole. This is the diseased liver pulse: When the pulse is full, replete, and slippery, it is the excess of a string-like pulse. Touching a long pole without the softness of its end means that the pulse is excessively string-like with scant stomach *qi*.

[10] When the pulse of the dying liver comes, it is as taut as touching the string of a drawn bow. This is the fatal liver pulse: The pulse is only string-like without stomach *qi*. So it is called the fatal liver pulse.

[11] When the pulse of the normal spleen appears, it is soft and natural as if a chicken walks in the field. This is the normal spleen pulse: A chicken walking in the field suggests that the pulse is graceful, light and slow, namely, slightly soft and weak with harmonious stomach *qi*.

[12] When the pulse of the diseased spleen comes, it is replete, full and rapid like a hen lifting its feet. This is the diseased spleen pulse: The pulse is replete, full and rapid. This suggests that the pulse loses its harmonious stomach *qi*. A hen lifts the feet; it means the pulse is light, rapid and not slow. So the spleen pulse is diseased.

[13] When the pulse of the dying spleen comes, it is sharp and hard like the beak of a crow or the claws of a bird, or it seems like the leakage of a roof or the flow of water. This is the fatal spleen pulse: The spleen *qi* is exhausted, so strange pulses appear. The pulse has not stomach *qi*, so it is the fatal spleen pulse.

[14] When the pulse of the normal kidneys appears, it is coherent, sleek, and slightly surging and full, and it is hard when touched. This is the normal kidney pulse: The pulse is coherent, slippery, and slightly surging and full like the heart pulse. The *yang* hides in the *yin*; it suggests that the pulse is slightly sinking.

[15] When the pulse of the diseased kidneys comes, it is as tight as a drawn vine and becomes harder when pressed. This is the diseased kidney pulse: The pulse is excessively sinking with scant stomach *qi*, so it is the diseased kidney pulse.

[16] When the pulse of the dying kidneys comes, it is as taut as touching a fiercely tugged rope, or solid as if the fingers are flicking at a stone. This is the fatal kidney pulse: Two men fiercely tug a rope against each other, or the fingers are flicking at a stone. This suggests that the pulse is only sinking without harmonious stomach *qi*.

6.4   Nineteenth Article

Discussion of Jade Arcana and Genuine Zang-Organs
The Plain Questions (excerpt)

6.4.1   Original article

"The genuine pulse of the liver feels taut both inside and outside. It is sharp and dreadful like touching the edge of a knife, or it is as taut as pressing the string of a musical instrument.[1] The patient's color is blue and white without gloss. The body hair falls off.[2] This condition means that the patient will die.

"The genuine pulse of the heart feels hard and short like touching the coix seeds.[3] The patient's color is red and black without gloss.[4] The body hair falls off. This condition means that the patient will die.

"The genuine pulse of the lungs feels large and vacuous. It seems as if feathers are put on the skin. The patient's color is white and red without gloss.[5] This condition means that the patient will die.

"The genuine pulse of the kidneys feels like it is beating fiercely. It is so solid as if the fingers are flicking at a stone. The patient's color is black and yellow without gloss.[6] The body hair falls off. This condition means that the patient will die.

"The genuine pulse of the spleen feels weak, suddenly rapid, and abruptly slow. The patient's color is yellow and blue without gloss.[7] The body hair comes off. This condition means that the patient will die.

"All patients with genuine pulses of the *zang*-organs will die."

The Emperor asked: "How can the expositions of the genuine pulses of the *zang*-organs lead to death?"

Uncle Qi answered: "The five *zang*-organs are all bestowed with *qi* by the stomach, which is the root of the five *zang*-organs. The *qi* of the *zang*-organs cannot reach the hand greater-*yin* lung channel. After being bestowed with the stomach *qi*, the *qi* of the *zang*-organs can reach the hand greater-*yin* lung channel.[8] So, the five *zang*-organs let their pulses be shown at the greater-*yin* lung channel at the corresponding seasons.[9]

"Therefore, when evils prevail, the essential *qi* will become feeble. Hence, in a serious case, the stomach *qi* cannot accompany the *qi* of a *zang*-organ to reach the hand greater-*yin* lung channel. So, the *qi* of this genuine *zang*-organ is exhibited alone. The lone exposition signifies the prevalence of evils. Thus it signifies death."

The Emperor said: "Marvelous!"

Commentary

This article describes the conditions of the genuine pulses of the *zang*-organs, and the reasons why they indicate death. It accentuates the significance of existence and exuberance of the stomach *qi*.

Annotation

[1] It is sharp and dreadful like touching the edge of a knife, or it is as taut as pressing the string of a musical instrument: This description reveals that the genuine pulse of the liver is string-like, thready and solid, namely, only string-like with absence of the stomach *qi*.

[2] The patient's color is blue and white without gloss. The body hair falls off: The blue color pertains to the liver. The white color indicates that metal torments wood. Because there is a fatal pulse, there must be fatal colors. The skin and body hair are glossy due to the nourishment of the defensive *qi*. If the body hair falls off, the defensive *qi* must have collapsed.

[3] Feels hard and short like touching the coix seeds: The coix seeds are short, replete and hard. This condition suggests that the pulse is not slightly surging and full.

[4] The patient's color is red and black without gloss: The color of fire is red, yet it has blackness without gloss. This suggests that water curbs fire. Therefore the patient will die.

[5] Feels large and vacuous. It seems as if feathers are put on the skin. The patient's color is white and red without gloss: The large and vacuous pulse means excessive exuberance. Feathers on the skin mean absence of root. The color of metal is white, yet it also has redness without gloss. This suggests that fire curbs metal.

[6] It is so solid as if the fingers are flicking at a stone. The patient's color is black and yellow without gloss: The pulse is only sinking without stomach *qi*. The black color pertains to water, yet yellow color accompanies it without gloss. This suggests that soil curbs water.

[7] Feels weak, suddenly rapid, and abruptly slow. The patient's color is yellow and blue without gloss: The *qi* of the *zang*-organ is so weak that the pulse is suddenly rapid and abruptly slow. The yellow color pertains to soil, yet the blue color concomitantly exists. This signifies that wood curbs soil.

[8] After being bestowed with the stomach *qi*, the *qi* of the *zang*-organs can reach the hand greater-*yin* lung channel: Showing at the wrist pulse.

[9] So, the five *zang*-organs let their pulses be shown at the hand greater-*yin* lung channel at the corresponding seasons: Such as the spring's string-like pulse, the summer's surging and full pulse, the autumn's floating pulse, the winter's sinking pulse, etc.

6.4.2   Original article

The Emperor said: "In all treatments, doctors should examine the appearance, *qi*, color and gloss, the exuberance or decline of the pulse, and whether it is a new or chronic illness. Then treatment can be adopted without delay.

"If the appearance is directly proportional to the *qi*,[1] the disease is curable. If the color is moist and iridescent, the disease is easy to cure. If the pulse is compliant with the season, the disease is curable. If the pulse is weak and slippery, it indicates that the stomach *qi* still exists, and the disease is easy to treat. Varying therapeutic methods should be used according to different seasons.

"If the appearance is inversely proportional to the *qi*, the disease is difficult to treat. If the color is lifeless and without gloss, the disease is difficult to cure. If the pulse is replete and solid, the disease is exacerbated. If the pulse is contrary to the season, the disease is not curable. The above-mentioned four difficulties[2] must be examined and the patient must be informed clearly."

Commentary

On the background of the integral idea that man and nature correspond, this article points out that in clinical diagnosis and treatment, a doctor must examine the patient's bodily appearance, spirit *qi*, color, gloss, pulse, etc., so as to predict an easy or a difficult recovery. The appearance is directly proportional to the *qi*. The color is moist and iridescent. The pulse is compliant with the season. The pulse is weak and slippery. These are the four easy conditions. The appearance is inversely proportional to the *qi*. The color is lifeless and without gloss. The pulse is replete and solid. The pulse is contrary to the season. These are the four difficulties. All the descriptions are meaningful in clinical practice and can determine prognosis.

Annotation

[1] If the appearance is directly proportional to the *qi*: The appearance is vigorous, while the *qi* is also exuberant; the appearance is weak, while the *qi* is also weak. If the appearance is vigorous, yet the *qi* is weak, or if the appearance is weak, yet the *qi* is exuberant, the disease will be difficult to treat.

[2] Four difficulties: The appearance is inversely proportional to the *qi*. The color is lifeless and without gloss. The pulse is replete and solid. The pulse is contrary to the season.

6.4.3   Original article

The Emperor said: "I was told that the vacuity and repletion can determine death and life. Please tell me about this condition."

Uncle Qi said: "The five vacuous signs determine death, and the five replete signs determine death as well. "

The Emperor said: "Go on."

Uncle Qi continued: "The excessive pulse, hot skin, abdominal distention, obstruction of the anterior and posterior orifices, and depression in the chest and dizziness, are the five signs of repletion. [1] The thready pulse, cold skin, scant *qi*, diarrhea and incontinence of urine, and inability of intake, are the five signs of vacuity. [2]"

The Emperor asked: "Why are there some people who survive?"

Uncle Qi answered: "If porridge enters the stomach and diarrhea stops, the patient with vacuity will survive. [3] If sweat and stool can be discharged, the patient with repletion will survive. [4] These are their symptoms."

Commentary

The five signs of repletion are the excess syndromes indicating that the five *zang*-organs are obstructed by evils. The situation will turn in their favor if "the sweat and stool can be discharged." This idea suggests that in the treatment of an excess syndrome, dispelling evils should be a priority adopted so as to allow the evils to exit, then the patient with repletion will survive. The five signs of vacuity are deficiency syndromes indicating that the essential *qi* of the five *zang*-organs is depleted. The situation will change in their favor if "porridge enters the stomach and diarrhea stops." So needless to say, this idea suggests that in the treatment of a deficiency syndrome, nourishing the stomach *qi* to cultivate the acquired basis is vitally important to the recovery of the essential *qi* of the five *zang*-organs.

Annotation

[1] The excessive pulse, hot skin, abdominal distention, obstruction of the anterior and posterior orifices, and depression in the chest and dizziness, are the five signs of repletion: The heart dominates the pulse. Since the pulse is excessive, the heart *qi* must be replete. The lungs dominate the skin and body hair. The skin is hot, so the lung *qi* is replete. The spleen dominates the abdomen. The abdomen is distended, so the spleen *qi* is replete. The kidneys open their windows at the anterior and posterior orifices. Their obstruction indicates that the kidney *qi* is replete. The liver opens its windows at the eyes. The depression in the chest and dizziness suggest that the liver

qi is replete.

[2] The thready pulse, cold skin, scant *qi*, diarrhea and incontinence of urine, and inability of intake, are the five signs of vacuity: The thready pulse indicates vacuous heart *qi*. The cold skin indicates vacuous lung *qi*. The scant *qi* denotes vacuous liver *qi*. Diarrhea and incontinence of urine indicate vacuous kidney *qi*. The inability of intake indicates vacuous spleen *qi*.

[3] If porridge enters the stomach and diarrhea stops, the patient with vacuity will survive: The *qi* of the five *zang*-organs is all produced by the stomach *qi*. When porridge gets into the stomach and diarrhea stops, the stomach *qi* is restored.

[4] If sweat and stool can be discharged, the patient with repletion will survive: Sweating indicates that the external repletion will be eliminated. Discharge of stool indicates that the internal repletion will be eradicated. The elimination of the external repletion causes the pulse to become harmonious and the hot skin to become cool. The elimination of the internal repletion enables the abdominal distention to disappear, the obstruction of the anterior and posterior orifices to become free, and the depression in the chest and the dizziness to terminate.

6.5   Forty-ninth Article

The Five Colors · The Divine Pivot (*excerpt*)

6.5.1   Original article

Lei Gong asked the Emperor: "Are the five colors singularly manifested in the Bright Hall?[1] I, young fellow[2] do not know what it means."

The Emperor answered: "The nose is called the Bright Hall. The area between the two brows is called the Watch-Towers at either Side of the Palace Gate. The forehead is called the Front Courtyard. The lateral cheek is called the Hedge. The tragus is called the Shield. These parts should be square, large and plump, and seen clearly beyond ten paces. Men with features like this will live to a hundred."

Lei Gong asked: "How do we examine the five sense organs?"

The Emperor answered: "The nasal bone is high, prominent, square and upright. The manifested parts of the five *zang*-organs are located orderly on the nose. The manifested parts of the six *fu*-organs display at both sides of the nose.[3] The manifested parts of the head and face are the area between the two brows and the forehead. The manifested part of the Imperial Palace (i. e., the heart) is at the Lower Extreme.[4] The five *zang*-organs stay calmly in the body. The true colors are exposed. The unhealthy colors are not exhibited. The nose is moist, glossy and clear. So the unfavorable conditions of the five sense organs can be detected."

Lei Gong asked: "Could you please tell me about the unfavorable conditions?"

The Emperor answered: "The five colors correspond to their own manifested parts. One whose manifested parts are sunken and not upright must suffer from illness. One in whose face a son's color exhibits at its mother's part[5] will not die even if the disease is serious."

Lei Gong asked: "How do the five colors dominate signs?"

The Emperor answered: "Blue and black dominate pain. Yellow and red dominate heat. White governs cold. These are the signs dominated by the five colors."

Lei Gong asked: "Some people die suddenly without disease. How can we know this?"

The Emperor answered: "He whose *zang-fu* organs are invaded by pernicious evils will die without disease."

Lei Gong asked: "Some people recover a little yet suddenly die. How can we know this?"

The Emperor answered: "Red color is exposed at the cheeks like a thumb in volume. Although the patient has recovered a little, he will die suddenly. Black color is exposed at the forehead like a thumb in volume. That man will die suddenly without disease."

Lei Gong bowed twice and said: "Magnificent! What about the death date?"

The Emperor answered: "Inspect the colors for prediction."

Commentary

This article discusses some types of color displayed in sudden death experiences, which are all summarized by ancient practitioners. They are worthy of further research.

Annotation

[1] The Bright Hall: i.e., the nose.

[2] I, young fellow: Lei Gong is the youngest one among all ministers. So he called himself as young fellow in a modest way.

[3] The manifested parts of the five *zang*-organs are located orderly on the nose. The manifested parts of the six *fu*-organs display at both sides of the nose: This content will be introduced and further explained in the following sections.

[4] The manifested part of the Imperial Palace (i.e., the heart) is at the Lower Extreme: The Lower Extreme is located at the mid-point between the two eyes. It is the manifested part of the heart. The heart is the monarch, so this manifested part is called the Imperial Palace.

[5] A son's color exhibits at its mother's part: Such as the yellow color shown at the part of the heart, the red color shown at the part of the liver, etc.

6.5.2　Original article

The Emperor said: "The forehead is the manifested part of the head and face. The upper part of the area between the two brows is the manifested part of the throat; the middle part of the area between the two brows is the manifested part of the lungs; the lower extreme[1] is the manifested part of the heart; the part just below the lower extreme, the liver; the left side of the liver, the gallbladder; the tip of the nose, the spleen; the alae of the nose, the stomach; the central parts between the alae of the nose and the cheekbones, the large-intestine; the outer sides of the large-intestine on the cheeks, the kidneys.

"The areas under the kidneys on the cheeks are the manifested part of the umbilicus; the parts between the nose and cheekbones above the nose-tip, the small-intestine; the philtrum, the bladder and womb; the parts of the cheekbones, the shoulders; the rear parts of the cheekbones, the arms; the parts below the arms, the hands; the areas just above the inner canthi, the chest and breasts; the parts just above the edges of the ears, the back; the parts along the gums below the *jiache* points,[2] the thighs; the central parts of the gums, the knees; the parts of the gums below the knees, the shins; the parts below the shins, the feet; the greater separation areas,[3] the inner sides of the thighs; the greater curve areas,[4] the patellae.

"The five *zang*-organs, six *fu*-organs, limbs and joints have their own manifested parts on the face. They have divisions of the *yin* and *yang*.[5] We should inspect them carefully, and discriminate between the left and right. This is called a great law of nature.[6] The manifested parts of color of an ill man are different from those of a woman. Those who master the *yin* and *yang* and carefully observe the gloss and gloom, are called proficient doctors."

Commentary

This article introduces in detail the manifested parts of color of the five *zang*-organs, six *fu*-organs and four limbs on the face in the color examination. It seems to imply the holographic idea in modern biology just like the acupuncture points of the ear lobes.

Annotation

[1] The lower extreme: The mid-point between the eyes.

[2] The *jiache* points: ST-6 who, i.e., Cheek Carriage.

[3] The greater separation areas: The soft muscle areas from the mouth corners to the *jiache* points.

[4] The greater curve areas: The two corners at both sides of the lower jawbone.

[5] They have divisions of the *yin* and *yang*: The left is *yang*, and the right is *yin*.

[6] We should inspect them carefully, and discriminate between the left and right. This is called a great law of nature: The left pertains to the *yang* and the right pertains to the *yin*. This idea conforms with the regularity of the opposites, *yin* and *yang*. Therefore, it is called a great law of nature.

6.5.3 Original article

"The deep and turbid facial colors indicate internal diseases. The floating and glossy facial colors indicate external diseases.[1] The yellow and red colors denote wind diseases. The blue and black colors denote pain.[2] The white denotes cold. The yellow with gloss of cream signifies pus.

"The excessive red signifies blood. The excessive pain may cause spasms. The excessive cold may incur numbness of the skin. The five colors are exposed at their own manifested parts. Inspect the floating or sinking to know a shallow ill place or a deep one. Inspect the gloss or gloom to predict a favorable prognosis or an unfavorable one. Check the dispersion or concentration to foretell a lengthy course or a short one.[3] Look at its being at the upper part or lower part to know an upper ill place or a lower one. Observe the facial colors with concentration to be aware of the past and now of a disease.

"Therefore, if a doctor fails to observe the patient's colors meticulously, he will not know the disease accurately. If the doctor is not distracted, he will understand the past and present conditions of the disease well. The color being bright, the disease is slight. The color being heavy and gloomy, the disease is serious. If the color is neither bright nor glossy, the disease is not quite bad. If the color is scattered like young horses galloping without congregation, and the scattered ill color is accompanied by pain due to *qi* stagnation, it suggests that the accumulation has not formed yet."

Annotation

[1] The deep and turbid facial colors indicate internal diseases. The floating and glossy facial colors indicate external diseases: If the facial color is deep, heavy, dreary, and gloomy, the disease is at the interior or *zang*-organs. If the facial color is light, floating, and glossy, the disease is at the exterior or *fu*-organs.

[2] The yellow and red colors denote wind diseases. The blue and black colors denote pain: The yellow and red are usually seen in wind-heat syndromes. The blue and black often coincide with stagnation of the *qi* and blood, so pain is reported.

[3] Check the dispersion or concentration to foretell a lengthy course or a short one: If the color is dispersed without gathering, the disease will be transient. If the color is focused without dismissal, the disease course will be prolonged.

6.6   Seventy-seventh Article

Discussion of Five Omissive Errors · The Plain Questions

6.6.1   Original article

The Emperor said: "Alas! The medicine is so immense and profound that it is like looking down into an abyss or greeting floating clouds. The abyss is still measurable, yet the floating clouds are boundless. The medical skills of sages are examples for people. The sages discussed and measured the minds of patients according to the laws. They obeyed the medical principles and rules strictly, practicing to serve people. So, doctors have five errors and four virtues in practice. Are you aware of them?"

Lei Gong left his seat and prostrated himself twice and said: "I am young, stupid, and perplexed. I did not hear about the five errors and four virtues. I can merely know them superficially, but fail in the access to their essentials. Sorry, I cannot offer a right answer."

The Emperor said: "In all diagnosis, doctors should ask the patient his past dignity and current obscurity. Although the patient has not been assaulted by evils, the disease occurs from within the body. It is called nutritive blood loss.[1] The patient was once rich, yet is now destitute. The disease is called essence loss.[2]

"The ill *qi* of the five *zang*-organs lingers, and it allies with the blood to induce diseases.[3] The doctor diagnoses with hesitation to determine the disease that is not at the *zang-fu* organs and does not change the body appearance. The disease name remains unknown as well. The patient becomes thinner and thinner. The *qi* becomes asthenic without essence. The disease is exacerbated with absence of the *qi*. The patient is often frightened with chills.[4] The disease is so deep, because his defensive *qi* is depleted outside and his nutritive blood is deprived inside. Even a good doctor may fail to understand the disease. This is the first error.

"In all diagnosis, doctors must ask diet and living, sudden joy and sudden bitterness, or past joy and current bitterness, which all can impair the essential *qi*. When the essential *qi* is exhausted, the body will collapse. Sudden anger damages the *yin*, and sudden joy damages the *yang*. The adverse *qi* moves upwards, the normal pulse loses its shape. An ignorant doctor does not know how to supplement and drain, and the true condition. The essence of the body is deserted day after day. The evils may attach to the *yin* or *yang* .[5] This is the second error.

"He who is skilled in pulse ought to perform classification and comparison,[6] and analyze concerned information unhurriedly. If a doctor does not apprehend this, his diagnosis will not be commendable. This is the third error.

"There are three routine inquiries[7] in practice. The doctor must inquire about the patient's dignity and obscurity, past high rank and current humbleness, and his desire for elevated status. If the patient was once dignified, yet is no longer, even if he is not invaded by evils, his spirit will be impaired inside, and the patient will be certain to perish. If the patient was once rich, yet is now indigent, although not assailed by evils, none the less his skin will wither, the tendons will bend, and atrophy, limp, and spasm will occur.[8]

"If the doctor cannot effectively persuade the patient to submit to instructions, such weak behavior will cause disorders and abnormalities. The disease will not be resolved, and the treatment will fail. This is the fourth error.

"In all practice, the doctor must know the onset and course of a disease. He must discriminate males from females in the pulse-taking. The emotional frustrations, such as loss of love, uncontrolled thought, melancholy, fear, joy and anger, may make the five *zang*-organs vacant, and make the blood and *qi* fail to act normally. However, the doctor cannot see such causes. How can we then say he has medical skills!

"The great blow due to a patient's loss of wealth may make his tendons seemingly severed and make his pulse seemingly disappearing. Though the body recovers movement, the fluids cannot be produced. The old wound becomes corrupt, and the *qi* and blood coagulate to produce heat. The heat attaches to the *yang* aspect, then the pus and blood amass to make the patient suffer intermittent chills and fevers. The untrained practitioner needles the *yin* and *yang* channels indiscreetly, so the body becomes slack and the four extremities become spasmodic. The death date will draw nigh.[9] If the doctor cannot understand the disease and determine its onset, and only predicts the death date, he is equally untrained. This is the fifth error. All the above five errors are committed by doctors who are not proficient in medicine and do not comprehend human matters."

Commentary

These segments enunciate in detail the five common mistakes committed by doctors in practice. They suggest that we should not only care for the common symptoms but also try to master the vicissitudes of patient's social life, and the changes of dignity, obscurity, poverty and wealth. The conditions of diet and living, the emotional state, the beginning and end of the disease, etc., should be interrogated as well. Only after the doctor inspects comprehensively, performs classification and comparison, and cares for pulse-taking, the five errors will be shunned. In the meantime, it is obvious that the article underscores the factors of emotional frustrations that may induce diseases. So in clinical practice, we should not ignore this condition.

Annotation

[1] It is called nutritive blood loss: It refers to depletion diseases due to emotional melancholy and thought.

[2] The disease is called essence loss: It refers to diseases due to essence loss caused by emotional frustrations.

[3] The ill *qi* of the five *zang*-organs lingers, and it allies with the blood to induce diseases: The nutritive blood loss and essence loss can all induce the *qi* of the five *zang*-organs to linger, then the disordered *qi* can ally with the blood to cause diseases.

[4] The disease is exacerbated with absence of the *qi*. The patient is often frightened with chills: The disease is deepened, and the *qi* is dispersed, so we say it is absence of the *qi*. The absence of the *qi* could induce deficient *yang*, so the patient is averse to cold. The deficient *yang* could bring about deficient spirit, so the patient is timid and often frightened.

[5] The evils may attach to the *yin* or *yang*: The doctor does not know how to supplement or drain, so that the *yin* and *yang* collapse. Hence, we say that the essence of the body is deserted day after day. When the *yang* is deserted, the evils attach to the *yin*; when the *yin* is deserted, the evils attach to the *yang*.

[6] Perform classification and comparison: To common diseases and uncommon ones.

[7] Three routine inquiries: Dignity or obscurity, poverty or wealth, and joy or bitterness.

[8] None the less his skin will wither, the tendons will bend, and atrophy, limp, and spasm will occur: The patient loses his fatty and sweet foods, then the fluids become dry, so atrophy, bending, limp, and spasm will occur. Furthermore, the melancholy and thought may impair the heart and lungs, then the *qi* and blood are damaged, so this disease will occur.

[9] The untrained practitioner needles the *yin* and *yang* channels indiscreetly, so the body becomes slack and the four extremities become spasmodic. The death date will draw nigh: The doctor does not know that the chills and fevers are due to the amassment of pus, thinking instead that they are symptoms of a common febrile disease, and rashly needles the *yin* and *yang* channels, further depleting the *qi*. So, the disease is exacerbated, the body becomes slack, and the four limbs become spasmodic. Eventually, the life is imperiled.

6.6.2 Original article

"Hence the saying: When sages treat diseases, they must know the heaven, earth, *yin* and *yang*, regularity of the four seasons, five *zang*-organs and six *fu*-organs, male and female, exterior and interior, acupuncture and moxibustion and healing stones, and functions of herbal remedies. They must cope with human matters unhurriedly in a common way of diagnosis. They must deal with the dignified, obscure, poor and wealthy people who have different moral characters and motivations. They must inquire about age, courage and fear, observe the colors and appearances of all body parts, comprehend the beginning and end of a disease, and consider the eight solar terms and nine portions of pulses.[1] The diagnosis must be thoughtful.

"As a law of treatment, inspecting original *qi* is most precious. If we fail to seek the disorder of the original *qi*, we should examine the exterior and interior for the source of the disorder, and then treat it. Adhere to the numbers to adopt treatment,[2] and do not disobey the theory of acupuncture. Being able to act according to these, a doctor will never fail in treatment. If the doctor does not know the theory of acupuncture, the five *zang*-organs may get heat stagnation and carbuncle may occur in the six *fu*-organs. A diagnosis without careful inspection is an abnormality. Strictly practice in accordance with the demands of medical classics, such as the *Upper Classic*, *Lower Classic*, *Surmising*, *Yin and Yang*, *Extreme Constancy*, and *Five Strokes*.[3] Observe the facial colors, and detect the beginning and end of a disease. Then, the doctor will be well-versed in any case."

Commentary

This article mainly talks about the four virtues. (1) The doctor must be aware of the changes of the heaven, earth, *yin*, *yang*, four seasons, and solar terms. (2) The doctor must comprehensively master medical knowledge of all branches. (3) The doctor must comprehend human matters. (4) The doctor must be good at diagnosis, make over-all analysis of a disease, and ascertain the pathology, so as to adopt proper treatments. All the above items are the basic medical virtues that any doctor should have, and the principles that any doctor should adhere to.

Annotation

[1] The eight solar terms and nine portions of pulses: The eight solar terms here refer to the Spring Equinox, the Autumn Equinox, the Summer Solstice, the Winter Solstice, the Beginning of Spring, the Beginning of Summer, the Beginning of Autumn, and the Beginning of Winter. The pulses of the whole body are divided into three parts — the head, arms and legs. The pulse of every part is further separated into three portions — the upper portion, middle portion, and lower portion. Therefore, there are nine portions of pulses in all.

[2] Adhere to the numbers to adopt treatment: Because the exterior, interior, *yin*, *yang*, *zang*-organs, *fu*-organs, and channels all have their normal numbers, so do not neglect these numbers.

[3] *Upper Classic*, *Lower Classic*, *Surmising*, *Yin* and *Yang*, *Extreme Constancy*, and *Five Strokes*: They are all ancient medical books, which are no longer extant.

Chapter Seven
Therapeutic Principles and Methods

Therapeutic principles are rules for treating diseases. These different therapeutic principles are based upon the integral idea, developed from pertinent data gathered by making the four examinations, and made according to the varying diseases or symptoms. These principles rely upon using different measures suited to different circumstances, different individuals, and different areas of the body; the tip and root; the moderation and urgency; the straight treatment and paradoxical treatment; warming cold and cooling heat, and so forth.

The therapeutic methods are concrete means to treat diseases following the directions of therapeutic principles according to different diseases or symptoms. A concrete method is ascribed to a concrete principle. For instance, the therapeutic principle of "discharging what is excess" includes therapeutic methods such as releasing the exterior, promoting vomiting (emesis), dispersing and leading, purgation, etc. The therapeutic principle of "supplementing what is weak" includes therapeutic methods such as enriching *qi*, moistening *yin*, warming *yang*, nourishing blood, etc.

In this chapter, some basic laws about herbal prescriptions are covered, which underlay the development of TCM prescriptions in later eras.

Therapeutic Principles and Methods

7.1   Seventy-fourth Article

Great Topic on Supreme Truth and Importance·
The Plain Questions (*excerpt*)

7.1.1   Original article

Cold is treated with heat. Heat is treated with cold. The slight is treated straight. The serious is treated paradoxically.[1] Hardness is whittled away.[2] Settling is treated by eliminating.[3] Fatigue is treated by warming.[4] Binding is treated by dissipating.[5] Lingering is treated by attacking.[6] Dryness is treated by moistening.[7] Spasm is treated by relaxing.[8] Scattering is treated by astringing.[9] Weakness is treated by warming.[10] Comfort is treated by moving.[11] Fright is treated by calming.[12] Raising, lowering,[13] massaging, bathing,[14] eroding, plundering,[15] opening,[16] or emanating[17] should be adopted to the disease in question.

Annotation

[1] The slight is treated straight. The serious is treated paradoxically: When a disease is slight, e.g., a *yang* disease shows heat, or a *yin* disease shows cold, warm what is cold or cool what is hot. This method is called straight treatment. When a disease is serious, (e.g., extreme heat engenders cold, or extreme cold engenders heat,) treat cold with cold, or treat heat with heat. This method is called paradoxical treatment.

[2] Hardness is whittled away: When there are hard accumulations or conglomerations inside the body, the method of whittling and attacking can be used.

[3] Settling is treated by eliminating: When evils intrude upon the body, we can expel them. For example, releasing the exterior to promote sweating can be used when evils lodge at the exterior; attacking interior to promote defecation can be used when evils lodge at the interior.

[4] Fatigue is treated by warming: Warming and tonifying can be used to asthenia due to fatigue.

[5] Binding is treated by dissipating: For stagnant *qi* and blood, phlegm or internal clumping of evil, dissipating method can be used.

[6] Lingering is treated by attacking: When pathogenic evil stays and does not retreat, such as lingering rheum, amassed blood, accumulated food, or stool obstruction, etc., attacking to defecate can be applied.

[7] Dryness is treated by moistening: Dryness syndrome with damaged fluids and water depletion can be treated by moistening and producing fluids.

[8] Spasm is treated by relaxing: The relaxing method can be used to treat spasms.

[9] Scattering is treated by astringing: Diseases with dissipation of the essential *qi*, such as spontaneous sweating or night sweating, can be treated by astringing.

[10] Weakness is treated by warming: Diseases with weakness and timidity can be treated by warming and tonifying.

[11] Comfort is treated by moving: When a man leads an excessively comfortable, sedentary lifestyle, the *qi* and blood may become stagnant, so moving the *qi* and quickening the blood circulation are appropriate treatment strategies.

[12] Fright is treated by calming: Settling the heart and mind can be adopted to heal the patient who is easily startled or fidgeted.

[13] Raising, lowering: When evils are at the upper part of the body, we can raise them through promoting vomiting (emesis). When evils are at the lower part of the body, we can try to lower them through purgation.

[14] Bathing: Using herbal decoction to wash, soak or rinse.

[15] Pplundering: Using drastic drugs to loot the evils.

[16] Opening: Opening orifices or opening to discharge, etc.

[17] Emanating: Emanating evils, lung *qi*, etc.

7.1.2   Original article

The Emperor asked: "What are straight treatment and paradoxical treatment?"

Uncle Qi answered: "Treating a disease straight is called a straight treatment.[1] Treating a disease paradoxically is called a paradoxical treatment.[2] The degree of straightness or paradoxicality is determined by the disease's degree."

The Emperor asked: "What is paradoxical treatment?"

Uncle Qi answered: "Treat heat with heat. Treat cold with cold.[3] Treat the obstructed by obstructing.[4] Treat the free by freeing.[5] The root of a disease must be treated and the cause of a disease must be sought. Their beginnings are identical, yet their ends are different.[6] Hence, accumulations can be dispersed, and the solidity can be broken. The *qi* can be harmonized, and the disease can be terminated.[7]"

The Emperor asked: "Fine. If one's *qi* is harmonious, yet he contracts a disease occasionally, how do you treat it?"

Uncle Qi answered: "Treat straight, or treat paradoxically, or straight first and then paradoxically, or paradoxically first and then straight, in order to dredge up the evils and make the *qi* harmonious. This is the policy."

Annotation

[1] Treating a disease straight is called a straight treatment: Treating heat with cold or treating cold with heat.

[2] Treating a disease paradoxically is called paradoxical treatment: Treating heat with heat or treating cold with cold.

[3] Treat heat with heat. Treat cold with cold: Use hot drugs to treat the syndrome of false heat and true cold. Use cold drugs to treat the syndrome of false cold and true heat.

[4] Treat the obstructed by obstructing: For example, the patient has weak *qi* at the lower part of the body, and the *qi* of the middle-warmer becomes stagnant. If you attack the obstruction first, fullness may be relieved a little when drugs get in; yet, fullness may subsequently return. The *qi* will become weaker, exacerbating the disease. In fact, taking little tonics will augment the fullness, yet taking more tonics can help to free the obstruction, and drastic tonics can completely dredge up the middle-warmer. Therefore, the lower deficiency is eliminated and the middle fullness is naturally dissipated. This is called treating the obstructed by obstructing.

[5] Treat the free by freeing: For example, a great heat accumulates inside, or a great cold congeals inside. The evil gathers and lingers to induce endless diarrhea. Discharge the congealed cold with hot drugs, or discharge the accumulated heat with cold drugs.

[6] Their beginnings are identical, yet their ends are different: Heat treats heat. Cold treats

cold. Obstructing treats the obstructed. Freeing treats the free. So, the beginnings are identical. At the end, the hot becomes cold, and the cold becomes hot. The obstructed becomes free, and the free becomes obstructed. So, the ends are different.

[7] Hence, accumulations can be dispersed, and the solidity can be broken. The *qi* can be harmonized, and the disease can be terminated: After obstructing treats the obstructed, the right *qi* is strengthened, which leads to dispersing the accumulation and breaking the solidity. After freeing treats the free, the evils are expelled. This condition leads to harmonizing the *qi* and ending the disease.

7.1.3 Original article

The Emperor asked: "It is known that cold is best treated with heat, and heat is best treated with cold. However, unlearned doctors are incompetent. They abolish the norm, and alter the principle. There is a heat disease, and the heat remains after being cooled. There is a cold disease, and the cold remains after being warmed. The old cold and heat still exist, yet new diseases arise again. How are they treated?"

Uncle Qi answered: "As to all that remains hot after being cooled, the *yin* should be selected.[1] As to all that remains cold after being warmed, the *yang* should be selected.[2] This is called seeking the essential attribute.[3]"

Commentary

These segments elucidate the straight treatment and paradoxical treatment, and the therapeutic principles of deficient heat and deficient cold. The straight treatment is namely the usual therapeutic method, which aims directly at the property and pathomechanism of a disease. The paradoxical treatment is employed, aiming at the superficial phenomenon of a disease.

With regard to the essentials of treatment, the nature of the used herbs is opposite to that of the manifested symptoms in both the straight treatment and paradoxical treatment. Therefore, the straight treatment and paradoxical treatment jointly obey the principles, i. e., "seeking the root of disease," "treating heat with cold, and treating cold with heat," and "draining what is excess, and supplementing what is deficient."

The deficient cold is caused by deficient *yang*, which produces external cold. The deficient heat is caused by deficient *yin*, which produces internal heat. The former shows cold signs, revealing that the deficient *yang* fails to warm. So the root of disease is deficient *yang*. The next shows heat signs, revealing the deficient *yin* fails to balance the *yang*. So the root of disease is deficient *yin*.

With regard to "seeking the root" and "supplementing deficiency and draining excess," the deficient *yang* should be selected when cold remains after warming treatment, and the deficient *yin* should be addressed when heat remains after cooling treatment.

"Nourishing *yin* to cool heat and supplementing *yang* to warm cold" when treating deficiency syndromes is completely different than "treating heat with cold and treating cold with heat" when treating excess syndromes. This dissertation outlines the therapeutic principles for cold syndrome and heat syndrome in clinical practice. It also underscores the significance in discriminating between deficiency and excess when diagnosing a heat or cold disease.

Annotation

[1] As to all that remains hot after being cooled, the *yin* should be selected: The deficient heat induced by *yin* deficiency cannot be cooled down by bitter and cold heat-discharging drugs. The method of supplementing *yin* should be used. The medical master, Wang Bing, referred to this as "strengthening the dominance of water to control the *yang* light."

[2] As to all that remains cold after being warmed, the *yang* should be selected: The deficient cold that is caused by *yang* deficiency cannot be expelled by pungent and hot cold-emanating drugs. It should be treated by the method of warming *yang*. Wang Bing referred to this as "boosting the source of fire to disperse the *yin* shadow."

[3] This is called seeking the essential attribute: i.e., inferring the *yin* or *yang* of a disease's attribute.

7.2   Twelfth Article

Discussion of Befitting Different Methods · The Plain Questions

Original article

The Emperor asked: "When doctors treat diseases, why are patients with similar diseases restored by different methods?"

Uncle Qi answered: "Landscapes make it so. The eastern area is where (the *yang qi*) of heaven and earth engenders.[1] That region teems with fish and salt, and has a long coast facing the sea. Its people eat fish and have a predilection for salt. The people are satisfied with their habitat and they feel all their foods to be delicious. Fish makes heat accumulate inside the body.[2] Salt may damage the blood.[3] Their skin is black and the muscular striae are loose. Their characteristic diseases are carbuncles and ulcers.[4] Healing stones are beneficial treatment.[5] Therefore, healing stones also come from the east.

"The west is an area abundant with gold, jade, sand and stone. (The *qi* of) heaven and earth is astringed here.[6] Its people live alongside windy hills where water and soil are rigid. The people wear coarse clothes, lie on hay mats, and eat greasy and fatty foods. So, evils cannot invade their bodies, yet diseases occur inside their body. Oral herbs are beneficial treatment.[7] Therefore, oral herbs also come from the west.

"The north is where (the *qi* of) heaven and earth is hold and stored.[8] The landscape is high, windy, chilly and icy. Its people are accustomed to wild roving and milk foods. The *zang*-organs are cold and fullness diseases occur.[9] Moxibustion is suitable treatment. So, moxibustion come from the north.

"The south is the area where everything grows and the *yang qi* is exuberant. The landscape is low. The water and soil are soft. Mist and dew converge there. Its people have a predilection for sour or fermented foods. Their muscular striae are loose and the skin is reddish. Their diseases are spasm and numbness.[10] The filiform needle is proper.[11] So, the nine needles also come from the south.

"The center has a flat and damp landscape, and living things are produced there in abundance by the heaven and earth.[12] Its people eat a wide variety of foods and are not overworked.[13] So, their diseases are commonly atrophy, *qi* reversal, and chills and fever.[14] *Qigong*[15] and massage are suitable. So, *qigong* and massage also originate from the center.

"Therefore, sages adopt a broad repertoire of methods to treat diseases,[16] yet every method is appropriate. So, although different methods are used, the patients all recover, because the sages recognize the causes of diseases and understand the major therapeutic methods."

Commentary

Any kind of different therapeutic method mentioned in these segments is summarized by people of east, south, west and north in practice. The different therapeutic methods have their suitable different diseases. Thus enlightened doctors consider the natural environments, individual differences, living customs, etc. They should master the therapeutic principles so as to take different measures to suit the time, place and the individual in question.

Annotation

[1] The eastern area is where (the *yang qi*) of heaven and earth engenders: The *yang qi* of heaven and earth rises from the east where is the beginning of the *yang qi*. The east corresponds to spring.

[2] Fish makes heat accumulate inside the body: Then carbuncles occur on the exterior of the body.

[3] Salt may damage the blood: Salty flavor runs to the blood. Excess salt produces thirst. Thirst due to excess salt is a sign of damaged blood.

[4] Their characteristic diseases are carbuncles and ulcers: The muscular striae are loose and the blood is weak, which allows carbuncles and ulcers to manifest in the skin, since the blood cannot nourish the skin properly.

[5] Healing stones are beneficial treatment: The diseases are at the skin. Healing stones are suitable to expel pus and blood in the skin layer.

[6] (The *qi* of) heaven and earth is astringed here: The *qi* of heaven and earth descends at the west, so it is astringed here. The west corresponds to autumn.

[7] Oral herbs are beneficial treatment: Diseases due to damage from diet and emotions occur at the interior. Acupuncture and massage will not be effective. So, only oral herbs are beneficial.

[8] The north is where (the *qi* of) heaven and earth is hold and stored: The north is chilly. It corresponds to the sign of holding and storing for winter.

[9] The *zang*-organs are cold and fullness diseases occur: The climate is chilly, and the property of milk is also cold, so the *zang*-organs become cold. There is much stagnation in cold *zang*-organs, so distention occurs.

[10] Their diseases are spasm and numbness: When the heat is overwhelming, the tendons be-

come spasmodic and dry. Mist and dew converge, and the damp wraps outside the body, so numbness occurs.

[11] The filiform needle is proper: There are nine kinds of needles in all. The filiform needle is appropriate for shallow needle techniques.

[12] The center has a flat and damp landscape, and living things are produced there in abundance by the heaven and earth: The body of soil is flat. It is damp in nature, and flourishes at the central part of the four directions. The soil is the mother of everything, so living things are abundant there.

[13] Its people eat a wide variety of foods and are not overworked: The center is the hub of the four directions. It is so prosperous and concentrated with people from all directions that the foods are varied and men have the luxury of time to rest.

[14] Their diseases are commonly atrophy, qi reversal, and chills and fever: The soil qi communicates with the spleen and dominates the four extremities. Thus, when the damp stagnates, atrophy occurs. When heat or cold exists, qi reversal occurs. The center is where the qi from the four directions converges, so it produces chills and fever.

[15] *Qigong*: A system of deep breathing exercise to regulate and reinforce the qi.

[16] Sages adopt a broad repertoire of methods to treat diseases: It means at some times, two or more therapeutic methods are combined to treat one disease.

7.3   Sixty-fifth Article

Discussion of Transmissions of Tip and Root Diseases ·
The Plain Questions （excerpt）

Original article

The Emperor asked: "What are the tip and root[1] of a disease? What are the straight needling and paradoxical needling?[2]"

Uncle Qi answered: "In all acupuncture practice, a doctor must differentiate between the *yin* and *yang*, and master the relationship between the first disease and the next one. He must take appropriate measures straight or paradoxically, and treat the tip and root flexibly.[3]

"So it is said that: The tip is treated when the disease is at the tip, or the root is treated when the disease is at the root, or the tip is treated when the disease remains at the root, or the root is treated when the disease remains at the tip. Therefore, the effect can be acquired by treating tip, or treating root, or straight treatment, or paradoxical treatment. Knowing the straightness and paradoxicality, a doctor can manipulate needles accordingly without needing to consult others; knowing the tip and root, a doctor can resolve all diseases; not knowing the tip and root is called reckless action.

"After apprehending the rules of the *yin*, *yang*, straightness, paradoxicality, tip and root, a doctor can comprehend diseases from the minor to the serious, and recognize the hazards of the hundred diseases when mentioning these rules. He can know diseases from little to many and from shallowness to profundity, and learn a hundred when speaking of one. These rules can help us discern the deep from the shallow and the distant from the near. The tip and root are easy to understand, yet difficult to practice.

"An erroneous treatment is unfavorable, and a right treatment is favorable[4] When a disease causes disorders (of the *qi* and blood), treat the root.[5] When disorders (of the *qi* and blood) cause a disease, treat the root. When cold produces a disease, treat the root. When a disease precedes cold, treat the root. When heat induces a disease, treat the root. When heat induces fullness of the middle-warmer, treat the tip.[6] When a disease produces diarrhea, treat the root. When diarrhea precedes disease, treat the root; the root must be regulated first, then the manifested disease is treated.[7]

"When a disease results in fullness of the middle-warmer, treat the tip. When the fullness of the middle-warmer results in vexation, treat the root.

"A man has new lodging evils and old lodged evils. When the urine and stool are inhibited, treat the tip.[8] When the urine and stool are smooth, treat the root. When a disease is excess, treat the root first, then treat the tip. When a disease is deficient, treat the tip first, then treat the root. Doctors should inspect the slightness and seriousness meticulously, and adjust the root and tip carefully. When a disease is slight, treat the tip and root simultaneously. When a disease is serious, treat the tip or root alone. When inhibited urine and stool bring about a disease, treat the root."

Commentary

These segments discuss the tip, root, straight needling and paradoxical needling, and enumerate the urgent and moderate treatments of the symptoms, such as diarrhea, middle fullness, vexation, and inhibition of urine and stool. The following therapeutic principles are explained: seeking the root in treatment; when the disease is urgent, treating the tip; when the disease is moderate, treating the root; and treating the tip and root simultaneously. The article sufficiently exhibits the propositions of aiming at the essence to treat diseases and of coping with concrete conditions flexibly.

Annotation

[1] The tip and root: As to a disease, the root is the fundamental cause of disease, and the tip is the clinical manifestations. As to two diseases involved, the root disease is the primary disease, and the tip disease is the secondary disease.

[2] The straight needling and paradoxical needling: For example, the disease is at the root and needle to treat the root, or the disease is at the tip and needle to treat the tip. This is called paradoxical needling. The disease is at the root and needle to treat the tip first, or the disease is at the tip and needle to treat the root first. This is straight needling.

[3] Treat the tip and root flexibly: In common conditions, when the disease is urgent, the tip should first be treated; when the disease is moderate, the root should first be treated. For example, a patient with usually weak *yang qi* is newly attacked by a common cold of wind-cold type with symptoms such as fever, headache, and a runny nose. A doctor should first treat the tip, i.e., the wind-cold symptoms. A patient with chronic headache due to flaming-up of deficient liver fire has additional symptoms such as chronic headache, afternoon (tidal) fever, thirst, and a bitter taste in the mouth. The root (deficient liver fire) should first be treated.

[4] An erroneous treatment is unfavorable, and a right treatment is favorable: If the doctor knows the root and tip, the treatment will be correct; not knowing the root and tip, the treatment

will be erroneous.

[5] When a disease causes disorders (of the *qi* and blood), treat the root: If a disease causes disorders of the *qi* and blood, the disease is the root and the disorders of the *qi* and blood are the tip.

[6] When heat induces fullness of the middle-warmer, treat the tip: As to all concerned pairs of diseases, the root should be treated first. Only for the fullness of the middle-warmer, the tip should be treated first, because the fullness suggests that evils are at the stomach. The stomach is the basis of the *zang-fu* organs. When the stomach is full, the *qi* of drugs cannot move, and the *zang-fu* organs fail to be nourished. So in this condition, the tip (fullness) should be treated first.

[7] When diarrhea precedes disease, treat the root; the root must be regulated first, then the manifested disease is treated: The root (diarrhea) is treated first. The diarrhea must make the middle soil deficient first. So, we should adjust and treat soil first, then treat the resulting disease. This process suggests we care for soil (spleen and stomach) first and foremost.

[8] When the urine and stool are inhibited, treat the tip: As to all concerned pairs of diseases, the root should be treated first. Only for the inhibition of urine and stool, the tip is treated first. Because the inhibition of urine and stool is a critical sign, so it must be treated first.

7.4   Fifth Article

Great Topic on Correspondences and Manifestations
of Yin *and* Yang· *The Plain Questions* (*excerpt*)

Original article

Hence the saying: When a disease begins, needling can stop it. When the disease is serious, wait till the disease wanes a little and then needle to stop it.[1] Thus, dissipate it according to its slightness.[2] Relieve it according to its seriousness.[3] Tonify it according to its debilitation.[4] When the form is insufficient, warm it with smells. When the essence is insufficient, supplement it with flavors.[5] The upper evils should be vomited.[6] The lower evils should be led and purged.[7] The middle fullness should be dispersed inside.[8] When there are evils, soak the patient to promote sweating.[9] When the evils are at the skin, promote sweating to emanate them. When the evils are fierce, restrain and control them. When a disease is replete, dissipate or discharge the evils.[10]

The doctor should inspect the *yin* and *yang*, and discern softness from rigidity. [11] When the *yang* is ill, treat the *yin*. When the *yin* is ill, treat the *yang*.[12] Stabilize the blood and *qi* of all channels, so that they can act in their normal positions. When the blood is replete, dredge it.[13] When the *qi* is weak, lift and enrich it.[14]

Commentary

This article asserts that in any treatment, the *yin*, *yang*, *qi*, blood, evil, right, deficiency and excess must first be distinguished. Doctors should adhere to the principles, such as dispelling evil and supporting right, supplementing deficiency and draining excess, replenishing essence in *yin* deficiency, warming *qi* in *yang* deficiency, treating *yang* in *yin* disease, treating *yin* in *yang* disease, etc. According to the lodging place of evils, such as the exterior, interior, upper part, middle part, or lower part, a different therapeutic method, such as releasing the exterior, vomiting, dispersing and leading, or purgation can be adopted. Furthermore, needling, oral administration, fuming, bathing, etc., are introduced. These discussions had a relatively great influence upon the development of therapeutic principle and therapeutic method in later eras, and upon the clinical practice as well.

Annotation

[1] When the disease is serious, wait till the disease wanes a little and then needle to stop it: In special conditions, the evils are so fierce that we had better not attack the evils directly. Wait the disease to wane a little and then needle to stop the disease.

[2] Dissipate it according to its slightness: The evils are slight and the disease is at the exterior, so dissipate the evils.

[3] Relieve it according to its seriousness: The disease is overpowering, so it is best to relieve it gradually in order to prevent the creation of an imbalance from an equally vigorous treatment.

[4] Tonify it according to its debilitation: When the evils recede, and the right *qi* becomes debilitated, tonification should be employed.

[5] When the form is insufficient, warm it with smells. When the essence is insufficient, supplement it with flavors: In speaking of form and essence, the form is *yang* and the essence is *yin*. In speaking of smells and flavors, the smells are *yang* and the flavors are *yin*.

[6] The upper evils should be vomited: The evils above the chest should be vomited.

[7] The lower evils should be led and purged: From urine or stool.

[8] The middle fullness should be dispersed inside: The evils cannot be vomited and purged, yet can only successfully be relieved by dispersing them inside the body.

[9] When there are evils, soak the patient to promote sweating: Soak the patient with herbal decoction, including steaming, fuming, soaking, bathing, etc.

[10] When a disease is replete, dissipate or discharge the evils: When the exterior is replete, dissipate the evils; when the interior is replete, discharge the evils.

[11] Discern softness from rigidity: The *yin* is soft and the *yang* is rigid. Discern the softness from rigidity, i.e., the *yin* from *yang*.

[12] When the *yang* is ill, treat the *yin*. When the *yin* is ill, treat the *yang*: When the *yang* is prevailing, the *yin* gets ill. When the *yin* is prevailing, the *yang* gets ill. For example, the *yin* of all that remains hot after being cooled should be selected; the *yang* of all that remains cold after being warmed should be selected.

[13] When the blood is replete, dredge it: Reducing blood stasis and letting bleeding are methods of dredging.

[14] When the *qi* is weak, lift and enrich it: For example, the Middle-tonifying Qi-Boosting Decoction is used to treat the sinking syndromes due to *qi* deficiency.

Principles of Formula Prescriptions

7.5   Seventy-fourth Article

Great Topic on Supreme Truth and Importance ·
The Plain Questions (excerpt)

7.5.1   Original article

The chief herb is called monarch. What assists the monarch is called minister. What responds to the minister is called envoy.

Commentary

Usually, a recipe is made of the monarch, minister, assistant and envoy. The monarch is the major one or two herbs with largest dosage by weight. The minister has relatively more kinds of herbs with relatively smaller dosage. The assistant and envoy have even smaller dosages. Their functions are roughly described as follows:

The monarch herb: It is the major one or two herbs aimed at the major disease or syndrome. The monarch herb is indispensable in a recipe.

The minister herb: It has two meanings. (1) One or more herbs helping the monarch to treat the major disease or syndrome. (2) One or more herbs providing the major therapeutic action to remedy the concurrent disease or syndrome.

The assistant herb: It has three meanings. (1) One or more assisting herbs that cooperate with the monarch and minister to strengthen the effect, or directly treat the secondary symptoms. (2) One or more assistance-controlling herbs used to moderate or eliminate the drastic or noxious properties of the monarch and minister. (3) One or more contrary-assistance herbs, which are contrary to the monarch in property. The herbs cooperate to treat the disease, when the disease is serious and the patient may refuse the drugs.

The envoy herb: It has two meanings. (1) One or more channel-leading herbs, which lead other herbs in the recipe to where the disorder manifests. (2) One or more harmonizing herbs, which coordinate and moderate other herbs in the recipe.

7.5.2   Original article

The Emperor asked: "One or more evils may exist. A disease may be serious or slight. A treatment may be moderate or urgent. A recipe may be big or small. What about their criteria?"

Uncle Qi answered: "The evils may lodge at the upper part or lower part. The disease may stay at the distant place or proximal place. The syndrome may be an interior one or an exterior one. The herbs may be heavy or light. However, it is the best to let herbs reach the diseased places.[1]

"The book *Great Importance* says: A recipe with a monarch and two ministers is an odd prescription;[2] two monarchs and four ministers, an even prescription;[2] two monarchs and three ministers, an odd prescription; two monarchs and six ministers, an even prescription. So we say: Make an odd prescription to a proximal disease. Make an even prescription to a distant disease. Do not make an odd prescription to promote sweating. Do not make an even prescription to discharge downward.[3] Supplement and treat the upper part with moderation. Supplement and treat the lower part with urgency.[4] Herbs with heavy smells and flavors should be used in an urgent case. Herbs with thin smells and flavors should be used in a moderate case. Let herbs penetrate to where the disease resides. That is just so. When a disease is at a distant place, avoid preventing herbs from reaching by food. Do not break the rule.[5]

"Therefore, the rule of harmonizing ill qi[6] is that: As to a proximal disease, an odd or even recipe with little amount of herbs should be prescribed; as to a distant disease, an odd or even recipe with large amount of herbs should be prescribed. A large recipe should have little kinds of herbs. A small recipe should have many kinds of herbs. The maximum can even reach nine kinds, and the minimum may even be two. If a disease cannot be defeated by an odd recipe, adopt an even recipe. That is called double recipe. If an even recipe cannot defeat a disease, try to use contrary-assistance herbs.[7] That is to say, cold, hot, warm and cool herbs are applied in a contrary way."

Commentary

This article discusses the basic principle of prescribing formulas. A formula includes the monarch, minister, assistant and envoy. It also presents the classifications of the large, small, urgent, moderate, odd, even, multiple and double prescriptions according to the disease degree, disordered place, urgent or moderate condition, odd number or even number of herbs, etc. The method of oral administration is also encompassed.

Annotation

¹ It is the best to let herbs reach the diseased places: Do not let the herbs to be surplus or insufficient.

² An odd prescription, an even prescription: An odd prescription is also called singular recipe with little herbs and special functions. An even prescription is also called multiple recipe with many herbs and wide functions.

³ Do not make an odd prescription to promote sweating. Do not make an even prescription to discharge downward: Only an even prescription is powerful enough to promote sweating. Only an odd prescription can discharge downward without attacking excessively due to toxic effects of herbs.

⁴ Supplement and treat the upper part with moderation. Supplement and treat the lower part with urgency: Moderate herbs can prevent evils from oppressing downward. Urgent herbs can prevent evils from settling in the middle-warmer.

⁵ When a disease is at a distant place, avoid preventing herbs from reaching by food. Do not break the rule: For example, when a disease is at the upper-warmer, take herb after dinner. When a disease is at the lower-warmer, take herb before dinner so that herbs are not stopped by food. This sentence suggests the time to take herb before dinner or after dinner.

⁶ The rule of harmonizing ill *qi*: The rule of making a prescription to harmonize ill *qi*.

⁷ Try to use contrary-assistance herbs: For example, add hot herbs in a cold recipe, or add cold herbs in a hot recipe.

7.6   Seventieth Article

Great Topic on Five Routine Rules · The Plain Questions (*excerpt*)

Original article

There are old diseases and new ones. There are large formulas and small ones. There are toxic herbs and non-toxic ones. So we should obey the routines to take herb. When greatly poisonous herbs are used to treat a disease, the treatment should be stopped when the disease is recovered sixty percent. When commonly poisonous herbs are used, the treatment should be stopped when the disease is recovered seventy percent. Slightly poisonous herbs, eighty percent. Non-poisonous herbs, ninety percent. Then, proper grains, meat, fruits and vegetables are taken to restore the health completely. Do not eat too much to impair the right *qi*. If the disease does not terminate, renew the above method.

Commentary

This article talks about the routine of taking herbs and the role of dietetic care. There are new diseases and old ones. There are large formulas and small ones. There are drastic and toxic herbs and mild ones. Therefore, although all herbs can be used to treat diseases, they may damage the right *qi*. So we should determine the degree of using herbs and the dietetic care, according to the drastic or mild property of herbs, and the degree of toxin. These are basic principles in clinical application even today.

Chapter Eight
Theory of Health Preservation

Health preservation means conserving vital power of one's life. The theory of health preservation deals with the theories, principles and methods of preserving health and prolonging life.

The theory of health preservation in *The Medical Classic of the Yellow Emperor* was formulated on the basis of the integral idea that man and nature are mutually corresponding. The theory apparently possesses the following characteristics.

(1) It puts the submission to nature as an important principle of health care. It maintains that "be submissive to the four seasons and adapt to cold and summer heat" and "be submissive to the climate and know the mysteriousness of nature." The principle of "nourishing the *yang* in spring and summer, and nourishing the *yin* in autumn and winter" is also underscored. If men are disobedient to the changes of the *yin* and *yang* of nature, disasters will follow; and diseases will not arise if men are obedient to them.

(2) One has to make adjustments of the mind and emotions since it is an important measure of health preservation. The theory asserts that men should "keep indifferent, tranquil, and cool to all desires," "accumulate the essence and protect the spirit," and "defend the spirit inside." So, the body form is not destroyed, and the spirit is not dissipated.

(3) The theory lays stress on the leading role to care the right *qi*. It regards that the right *qi* exists inside, and evils cannot make disturbance, and also points out that protecting and strengthening the right *qi* should be the basic principle behind all methods of health care. If our actions are consistent with this principle, the destination that "strange evils will not come and longevity could be acquired" will be reached.

8.1   First Article

Discussion of Heavenly Truth in Ancient Times ·
The Plain Questions

8.1.1   Original article

In ancient times, the Yellow Emperor was very clever after born. As a baby, he learned to speak before the others could. In his childhood he was thoughtful. The Emperor was honest and shrewd in his youth, and mounted the throne since he was grown-up.

The Emperor asked Uncle Qi: "I was told all the remote ancients lived over a hundred years, yet their movements were still vigorous. However, the nowaday people become debilitated in their movements when they are only fifty. Have the times changed? Or, do people fail to exercise the health care?"

Uncle Qi answered: "The remote ancients who had the knowledge of health care followed the canons of the *yin* and *yang*, practiced physical exercises appropriately,[1] and had temperate diets. They led regular lives, and did not work against the routine. Therefore, their body forms co-existed with the spirits, and they could enjoy their natural ages and only died after they were a hundred.

"However, our nowaday people do not behave like these. They take wine as beverage, lead an abnormal life as a routine, and make love when being drunken. Their essence is exhausted by desires, and their genuine *qi* is dissipated by the favorite things. They do not know how to keep the essential *qi* full, and are not good at regulating their spirits. Yet, they hanker after a moment's pleasure against the funs of health care, and lead irregular lives. Therefore, these people are feeble in their fifties."

Commentary

This section points out that the remote ancients adhered to the rules of health preservation and lived to a hundred years; the nowaday people disobey the rules of health care and become feeble even when they are fifty. It suggests that man's life-span is not determined by the differences of times, but depends on the fact whether he follows health care or not.

It is apparent that health care is very significant towards prolonging life. The original article presents the principles of health care, such as following the canons of the *yin* and *yang*, taking appropriate physical exercises, having temperate diets, leading a regular life, making love with austerity, using propriety in work and rest, conserving the body essence, keeping the mind tranquil, etc. All these ideas form the basis for the theory of health preservation in TCM.

Annotation

[1] Practiced physical exercises appropriately: Including leading the *qi*, massage, breathing, etc.

8.1.2 Original article

"The remotely ancient sages instructed people to follow the rules of health preservation. Evaded the weakness-attacking evils and bandit wind with a due consideration to the time.[1] Kept indifferent, tranquil, and cool to all desires. Harmonized the genuine *qi*, and defended the spirit inside. Then, where could diseases come from?

"Thus, people had calm and care-free minds with little desires. Their hearts were restful without fears. Their bodies were overworked, yet without fatigue. Their genuine *qi* was harmonious and smooth. What they desired could be acquired, and what they anticipated could be obtained.[2] So, people felt their foods delicious, their clothes comfortable, and their customs gleeful. The superiors and inferiors were satisfied with their status. The people were just as plain as this.

"Thus, their favorites and desires could not disturb their vision. Lascivious evils could not infatuate their hearts. The stupid, intelligent, sagacious or vulgar men were not bothered by things. Thus they were submissive to the norms of health preservation. Therefore, the reason why they had vigorous movements even at the age of over a hundred was that they had perfected health cares, and senility could not threaten them."

Commentary

In the natural circumstance, we should evade the weakness-attacking evils and bandit wind with a due consideration to the time. As to the body, we should keep indifferent, tranquil, and cool to all desires, and defend the spirit inside. In this way, we can make the genuine *qi* harmonious and no disease will occur. The viewpoints of caring for the essence and *qi* and spirit, and of vigorously resisting against exogenous evils, are the leading ideas behind disease prevention and health care in TCM.

Annotation

[1] The weakness-attacking evils and bandit wind: Evils enter the weak points of the body, so they are called weakness-attacking evils. Here, the weakness-attacking evils and bandit wind refer to all pathogenic evils.

[2] What they desired could be acquired, and what they anticipated could be obtained: Because their desires were small and few.

8.1.3 Original article

The Emperor asked: "An old man (woman) becomes infertile. Is his (her) reproductive ability used up? Or, is the cause of his (her) natural age?"

Uncle Qi answered: "When a female is seven years old, the kidney *qi* prevails. The teeth change, and the hair grows. When she is fourteen years old, the reproductive material is produced. The controlling channel opens. The penetrating channel turns exuberant. The menstruation comes regularly, so she can bear a child. At the age of twenty-one, the kidney *qi* is full. So, the wisdom teeth appear, and she reaches her maturity. At the age of twenty-eight, the tendons and bones are solid. The hair is long, and the body is prosperous and strong. At the age of thirty-five, the bright-*yang* stomach channel wanes. The face begins to wither, and the hair begins to fall.[1] At the age of forty-two, the three *yang* channels become feeble at the upper part of the body. The face withers, and the hair turns grey. At the age of forty-nine, the controlling channel becomes debilitated, and the *qi* and blood of the penetrating channel decline and become scanty. The reproductive material is exhausted, and the menstrual tunnel becomes obstructed. As the body form is destroyed greatly, a woman becomes infertile.

"When a boy is eight years old, the kidney *qi* becomes replete. The hair grows, and the teeth change. At the age of sixteen, the kidney *qi* is exuberant, and the reproductive material is produced. The essential *qi* is full and leaks.[2] The *yin* and *yang* are harmonious, so he can father a child. At the age of twenty-four, the kidney *qi* is full, and the tendons and bones are strong and powerful. Thus, the wisdom teeth appear, and he reaches his maturity. At the age of thirty-two, the tendons and bones are prominent and prosperous, and the muscles are full and strong. At the age of forty, the kidney *qi* is declining. The hair falls, and the teeth wither. At the age of forty-eight, the *qi* of the three *yang* channels is exhausted at the upper part of the body. The face withers, and the hair is grey. At the age of fifty-six, the liver *qi* begins to decline, and the tendons cannot move. At the age of sixty-four, the reproductive material is depleted. The essence is scanty, and the kidneys are feeble. The body form is entirely debilitated, and the teeth and hair disappear. The kidneys dominate water.[3] They receive the essential *qi* of the five zang-organs and six fu-organs and store it. So only when the five zang-organs are prosperous, the kidneys are able to discharge seeds. Now, the five zang-organs are all feeble. The tendons and bones are slouchy. The reproductive material is used up. Thus, his hair becomes grey, the body is cumbersome; he hobbles and becomes infertile."

The Emperor asked: "Why can some old people have children?"

Uncle Qi answered: "Because they have extraordinarily long ages. The qi and blood of channels are still free, and the kidney qi is in surplus. Though being able to have a child, a man will not be more than sixty-four, and a woman will not be older than forty-nine, when their essential qi is completely exhausted."

The Emperor asked: "Can people still have children, who are knowledgeable of taking care of their health and are older than a hundred?"

Uncle Qi answered: "People skilled in health care can prevent senility and preserve their bodies. Though very old, they are still fertile."

Commentary

This article mainly discusses the relationship between the kidney qi and the growth and fertility. The article points out that the growth and fertility of a man are mainly determined by the kidney qi, so the important role of the kidneys in the whole life's activities is exhibited so eminent here. Because the essential qi of the kidneys is directly pertinent to growth and senility, so the crucial point of health care lies in protecting and preserving the essential qi.

The exuberance or decline of the kidney qi is also related to a person's sexual ability and reproductive ability. This academic idea had a far-reaching influence upon the clinical medicine in later eras. For instance, the relationship between the penetrating channel and controlling channel, and the menstruation and reproduction became the basis for the development of gynecology in later periods of time. This theory is also the reference to treatments of male impotence, seminal emission, sterility, etc.

Annotation

[1] The bright-yang stomach channel wanes. The face begins to wither, and the hair begins to fall: The bright-yang stomach channel has copious qi and blood. When it wanes, the qi and blood fail to nourish the skin pores, so the hair begins to fall. The bright-yang channel runs through the face, so the face begins to wither.

[2] The essential qi is full and leaks: The semen is full and leaks naturally.

[3] The kidneys dominate water: It implies that the kidneys store the essence.

8.1.4 Original article

The Emperor said: "I was told that there existed genuine men in the remotely ancient times. They mastered the rules of the heaven, earth, *yin* and *yang*, and inhaled and exhaled the essential *qi* of nature.[1] They independently defended the spirits inside, and kept the skin and muscles vigorous all the time. So their longevity could compete with that of the heaven and earth and their lives had no end. This was the outcome of perfect health preservation.

"There were supreme men in the middle ancient times who possessed upright virtues and skilled health care. They adapted themselves to changes of the *yin*, *yang* and four seasons. Staying above the secular world, they accumulated the essences and protected the spirits. Their thoughts roamed between the heaven and earth, and their watching and listening reached the eight directions. Because of this they prolonged their lives and strengthened their bodies following the genuine men.

"Secondly, there were also sages. They lived in harmony with the heaven and earth, and submitted to the rules of the eight winds.[2] They adapted their hobbies and desires to the ordinary world, and did not harbor any anger and resentment. Their behaviors and thoughts were away from the vulgar people, although living in the ordinary world. Their bodies were not fatigued by matters outside. Their minds were not perturbed inside. They kept tranquil, optimistic and self-contented. Their bodies were not destroyed. Their essences and spirits were not dissipated. Their life-span could also reach a hundred years.

"Next, there were sagacious men. They followed the rules of the heaven and earth, acted in accordance with the running of the sun and moon, and ascertained the changes of the stars. The sagacious men submitted to the *yin* and *yang*, and differentiated the four seasons. They practiced following the remotely ancient people, and adhered to rules of health preservation. Their life-span was also prolonged to the boundaries of its natural limitation."

Commentary

The four kinds of masters of health preservation — genuine man, supreme man, sage, and sagacious man are idealistic exemplars in the thoughts of the authors of *The Medical Classic of the Yellow Emperor*, not concrete individuals. The goal of introducing these four kinds of men is to explain that different ways and degrees of health preservation would result in differing effects.

Annotation

[1] Iinhaled and exhaled the essential *qi* of nature: e.g., exercised the *qigong*.

[2] They lived in harmony with the heaven and earth, and submitted to the rules of the eight winds: It means adapting to all climatic changes. The eight winds are namely winds from the east, south, west, north, southeast, northeast, southwest, and northwest.

8.2   Second Article

Great Topic on Adjusting Spirit According to Qi
of the Four Seasons · The Plain Questions

8.2.1   Original article

The three months of spring[1] are called generation and staleness elimination.[2] The lively *qi* of the heaven and earth is growing, and everything is
flourishing. A man should go to bed late and get up early. Stroll slowly in the
garden, loosen the hair and relax the body, so as to let thoughts act vigorously.[3] He should make things alive not dead, give things to others and not deprive others of things, and reward others rather than punish.[4] These behaviors
are respondences to the spring *qi*, and ways of nourishing generation. If he is
disobedient to these, the liver will be impaired, and a cold disease will occur
in the summer, because of a bad basis for summer growth.[5]

The three months of summer[6] are called exuberance and beauty. The
heavenly *qi* and earthly *qi* cross,[7] and everything blooms and bears fruits. A
man should go to bed late and get up early, and not be abhorrent of sunshine,[8] so as to turn away his mind from anger, and let his spirit become vigorous and let the *yang qi* discharge to the outside, just as if his beloved things
were at the outside.[9] These behaviors are respondences to the summer *qi*, and
ways of nourishing growth. If he is disobedient to these, the heart will be
damaged, and malaria will occur in the autumn,[10] because of a bad basis for
autumn harvest.

The three months of autumn[11] are appearance stability.[12] The heavenly
qi[13] is swift and harsh, and the colors of the earth are solemn and clear. A
man should sleep early and get up early with the cocks, so as to make the
mind calm and to moderate the torment of the harsh autumn *qi*. He should astringe the spirit to make the autumn *qi* safe for him, and should not expose
his mind so as to make the lung *qi* clear. These behaviors are respondences to
the autumn *qi*, and ways of nourishing harvest. If he is disobedient to these,
the lungs will be hurt, and diarrhea containing undigested foods will occur in
the winter, because of a bad basis for winter storage.

The three months of winter[14] are called blockage and storage. The water is frozen and the earth is cracked. The *yang qi* of nature is stored without disturbance. A man should sleep early, and get up late when the sun shines, so as to make his mind seemingly hidden, as if he had private thoughts or has acquired a thing. Evade cold and approach warmth.[15] Do not sweat excessively to render his *yang qi* frequently depleted. These behaviors are respondences to the winter *qi*, and ways of nourishing storage. If he is disobedient to these, the kidneys will be spoilt, and atrophy and *qi* reversal diseases will occur in the spring,[16] because of a bad basis for spring generation.

Commentary

This section points out that men should preserve health according to the regularity of the spring generation, summer growth, autumn harvest and winter storage, so as to adjust the spirit and mind, prevent diseases, and keep healthy. These ideas embody the integral idea that man and nature are mutually corresponding, and explain that the thought of disease prevention and the ways of health preservation cannot be separated in TCM.

Annotation

[1] The three months of spring: Including the Beginning of Spring, Rain Water, Wakening of Insects, Spring Equinox, Pure Brightness, and Grain Rain.

[2] Generation and staleness elimination: In spring, the *yang qi* has increased. Everything is growing and new, while stale things are eliminated.

[3] A man should go to bed late and get up early. Stroll slowly in the garden, loosen the hair and relax the body, so as to let thoughts act vigorously: Along with the lively spring *qi*.

[4] He should make things alive not dead, give things to others and not deprive others of things, and reward others rather than punish: In spring, one's thoughts and activities should be obedient to the lively generating *qi* of spring. So we should make things alive, give things to others and reward others, yet we could not make things dead, deprive others of things and punish others.

[5] If he is disobedient to these, the liver will be impaired, and a cold disease will occur in the summer, because of a bad basis for summer growth: The liver pertains to wood and dominates spring. If he is disobedient to the spring *qi*, the liver will be damaged. Wood is impaired and fails to engender fire. So, a cold disease will occur in the summer, and the basis for summer growth is bad.

[6] The three months of summer: Consisting of the Beginning of Summer, Lesser Fullness of Grain, Grain in Beard, Summer Solstice, Lesser Heat, and Greater Heat.

[7] The heavenly *qi* and earthly *qi* cross: The *yin qi* and *yang qi* wane or wax, and they cross in summer. So, we say that the heavenly *qi* and earthly *qi* cross in summer.

[8] Not be abhorrent of sunshine: A man is apt to be abhorrent of the long sunshine in the summer. However, the summer dominates the growth of the *qi*, so do not detest the long sunshine.

[9] The *yang qi* discharge to the outside, just as if his beloved things were at the outside: Let

the *yang qi* diffuse and spread at the body surface just as if his beloved things were at the outside, so as to adapt to the circumstance with the flourishing *yang qi*.

[10] The heart will be damaged, and malaria will occur in the autumn: The heat overrides the heart. When the autumn comes, the autumn *qi* is astringent, while the heat is stagnant inside the body. Thus, the *yin* wants to enter, yet the *yang* repels it; the fire wants to get out, yet the *yin* binds it. Therefore, the metal and fire fight each other, and fevers and chills go to and fro intermittently.

[11] The three months of autumn: Involving the Beginning of Autumn, End of Summer, White Dew, Autumn Equinox, Cold Dew, and Frost's Descent.

[12] Appearance stability: The appearances of all things are stable.

[13] The heavenly *qi*: Here refers to the wind.

[14] The three months of winter: Comprising the Beginning of Winter, Lesser Snow, Greater Snow, Winter Solstice, Lesser Cold, and Greater Cold.

[15] Evade cold and approach warmth: To nourish the *yang qi*.

[16] Atrophy and *qi* reversal diseases will occur in the spring: The damaged kidneys fail to promote the liver that dominates the tendons, so atrophy occurs in the spring. The *yang qi* is not well stored in the winter, so the *yang qi* is deficient, and *qi* reversal occurs.

8.2.2   Original article

The heavenly *qi* is clear and bright. The heaven conceals virtues and runs endlessly. So, the heaven will never fall. If the heaven is murky, then the sun and moon are not bright, and evils may poison the space between the heaven and earth.

The heavenly *yang qi* is blockaded, and the earthly *yin qi* is dim.[1] The clouds and fogs do not brighten. So, the white dew of the heaven does not descend correspondingly,[2] and the communication is not harmonious.[3] The lives of all things lose their endowment, and most famous trees die.[4] The noxious evils devastate nature greatly. The winds and rains are not moderate. The white dew does not descend. So, even luxuriant trees and paddy rice stalks cannot flourish. The bandit wind comes frequently. The torrential rains usually pour down. The natural four seasons cannot preserve their normal variations.

If a man acts disobediently to the rules of health preservation in this situation, he will die in the midst of his normal life-span. Only sages submit themselves to the rules of health care, so they will not contract strange diseases. They live harmoniously with all things, so their vitality will not be exhausted.

Commentary

This article explains that the variations of climates directly affect the flourishing, withering, life and death of all living things, so as to persuade men to take care of health with obedience to climatic changes. In this way, the vital *qi* can be preserved, and the longevity can be acquired. Otherwise, man will contract diseases or perish.

Annotation

[1] The heavenly *yang qi* is blockaded, and the earthly *yin qi* is dim: The evils poison the space. So, the heavenly *yang qi* is blockaded and fails to descend, and the earthly *yin qi* is dim and fails to ascend.

[2] The clouds and fogs do not brighten. So, the white dew of the heaven does not descend correspondingly: The earthly *qi* ascends to be clouds and fogs. If the earthly *qi* does not ascend, then the clouds and fogs do not brighten. The heavenly *qi* descends to be rains and dew. If the heavenly *qi* does not descend, then correspondingly the white dew does not descend.

[3] The communication is not harmonious: If the heavenly *qi* descends and the earthly *qi* ascends, a harmonious communication is formed.

[4] Most famous trees die: In this situation, big trees die, let alone other living things.

8.2.3   Original article

If one is disobedient to the spring *qi*, the *qi* of the lesser-*yang* will not be generated, and the liver *qi* will change inside.[1] If one is disobedient to the summer *qi*, the *qi* of the greater-*yang* will not grow, and the heart *qi* will be vacant inside.[2] If one is disobedient to the autumn *qi*, the *qi* of the lesser-*yin* will not be harvested, and the lungs will be wizened with fullness.[3] If one is disobedient to the winter *qi*, the *qi* of the greater-*yin* will not be stored, and the kidney *qi* will sink alone.[4] The *yin* and *yang* of the four seasons are the root of all things.

Therefore, sages nourish the *yang* in spring and summer, and nourish the *yin* in autumn and winter,[5] so as to obey the root. Thus, the sages perpetually resonate with all living things in the course of life. If one is disobedient to this root, the basis of life will be attacked, and his genuine *qi* will be destroyed. Therefore, the *yin* and *yang* of the four seasons are the beginning and end of all things, and the root of death and life. If one is disobedient to this, disasters will ensue; if one is obedient to this, diseases will not arise. It is called attainment of the rules of health preservation. As to the rules of health preservation, sages fulfill them, yet the stupid disobey them. Being obedient to the *yin* and *yang* means life; being disobedient means death. If one is obedient to this, the disease will be curable; if one is disobedient, the condition will be disordered. If one disobeys this rule, the caused disease is called internal repellence.[6]

Thus, the sages do not treat a formed disease, but treat an unformed disease;[7] they do not treat a formed disorder, but treat an unformed disorder. That is just so. If medicines are only used once a disease has formed, or treatments are only taken when a disorder has formed, this condition is just like digging a well when one is thirsty, or like casting knives when one is about to fight. It is late, isn't it?

Commentary

The *yin* and *yang* of the four seasons are the root of all things. This tenet penetrates through the whole article. It is not only the theoretical basis for the integral idea that "man and natue are mutually corresponding" in *The Medical Classic of the Yellow Emperor*, but also the important theoretical pillar of the theory of health preservation in TCM.

The original article underscores the importance of nourishing the *yang* in spring and summer, and nourishing the *yin* in autumn and winter. This viewpoint is the very significant principle of health care in the four seasons. Only when people are obedient to changes of the four seasons to preserve health that they can efficiently prevent disease and prolong life. This article also presents the proposition of curing unformed diseases, embodying the thought of disease prevention in TCM sufficiently.

Annotation

[1] If one is disobedient to the spring *qi*, the *qi* of the lesser-*yang* will not be generated, and the liver *qi* will change inside: The liver dominates spring, and spring dominates generation. If one is disobedient to the spring *qi*, the *qi* of the lesser-*yang* will not be generated. The liver *qi* will be stagnant, and liver disease will occur.

[2] If one is disobedient to the summer *qi*, the *qi* of the greater-*yang* will not grow, and the heart *qi* will be vacant inside: If one is disobedient to the summer *qi*, the *yang* will not be exuberant, and the heart *qi* will be vacant inside.

[3] If one is disobedient to the autumn *qi*, the *qi* of the lesser-*yin* will not be harvested, and the lungs will be wizened with fullness: If one is disobedient to the autumn *qi*, the *qi* of the lesser-*yin* will fail to be astringent, and the lung *qi* will be uneven.

[4] If one is disobedient to the winter *qi*, the *qi* of the greater-*yin* will not be stored, and the kidney *qi* will sink alone: If one is disobedient to the winter *qi*, the *qi* of the greater-*yin* will fail to be stored, and the kidney *qi* will leak downward.

[5] Sages nourish the *yang* in spring and summer, and nourish the *yin* in autumn and winter: Nourish the generation and growth in spring and summer, and nourish the harvest and storage in autumn and winter.

[6] If one disobeys this rule, the caused disease is called internal repellence: The movements of the *qi*, blood and *zang-fu* organs in the body are not harmonious with the changes of *yin* and *yang* of nature.

[7] The sages do not treat a formed disease, but treat an unformed disease: Treat a disease before it occurs. Prevent a disease from occurring.

Appendix

Chinese Equivalents for Some Important Terms

黄帝	the Yellow Emperor
歧伯	Uncle Qi
天人相应	nature and man are mutually corresponding
阴阳	*yin*, *yang*
表里	exterior, interior
寒热	cold, heat
虚实	vacuity, repletion (deficiency, excess)
木火土金水	wood, fire, soil, metal, water
怒喜思悲恐	anger, joy, thought, sorrow, fear
酸苦甘辛咸	sour, bitter, sweet, acrid, salty
风热湿燥寒	wind, heat, damp, dryness, cold
爪面唇毛发	nails, face, lips, body hair, hair
筋脉肉皮骨	sinews, vessels, flesh, skin, bones
生长化收藏	generation, growth, bloom, harvest, storage
相生	inter-promotion
相克	inter-curb
相乘	inter-overcontrol
相侮	inter-insult
五脏	five *zang*-organs
心肺	heart, lungs
肝脾肾	liver, spleen, kidneys
六腑	six *fu*-organs
小肠大肠胃	small-intestine, large-intestine, stomach
胆囊膀胱	gallbladder, bladder
三焦	triple-warmer
上焦	upper-warmer
中焦	middle-warmer
下焦	lower-warmer

脏象	*zang*-organs and manifestations
奇恒之腑	extremely constant *fu*-organ
腠理	muscular striae
胁	rib-side
气	*qi*
血	blood
津	liquid
液	fluid
营气(营血)	nutritive *qi* (nutritive blood)
卫气	defensive *qi*
宗气	ancestral *qi*
精	essence
神	spirit
魂	*yang* soul
魄	*yin* soul
意	idea
志	resolution
髓海	sea of marrow
血海	sea of blood
气海	sea of *qi*
水谷之海	sea of water and grains
魄门	anus
鬼门	ghost gate (sweat pores)
净腑	clear *fu*-organ (bladder)
经络	channels and network-channels
寸口脉	wrist pulse
寸	thumb-width
人迎脉	neck pulse
手阳明大肠经	hand bright-*yang* large-intestine channel
手少阳三焦经	hand lesser-*yang* triple-warmer channel
手太阳小肠经	hand greater-*yang* small-intestine channel
手少阴心经	hand lesser-*yin* heart channel
手厥阴心包经	hand cold-*yin* pericardium channel
手太阴肺经	hand greater-*yin* lung channel
足阳明胃经	foot bright-*yang* stomach channel
足少阳胆经	foot lesser-*yang* gall-bladder channel

足太阳膀胱经	foot greater-*yang* bladder channel
足少阴肾经	foot lesser-*yin* kidney channel
足厥阴肝经	foot cold-*yin* liver channel
足太阴脾经	foot greater-*yin* spleen channel
督脉	governing channel
任脉	controlling channel
冲脉	penetrating channel
带脉	girdling channel
阴维脉	*yin*-linking channel
阳维脉	*yang*-linking channel
阴跷脉	*yin*-springing channel
阳跷脉	*yang*-springing channel
井穴	exit point
荥穴	slip point
输穴	inrush point
经穴	pass point
合穴	entrance point
背腧穴	back transport point
募穴	converging point
补	supplement（tonify）
泻	drain（discharge）
鱼际	fish-abdomen-style muscles
髀	hip
巅	vertex
颃颡	palate
畜门	nostrils
篡	perineum
跗	instep
眦	canthus
尻	buttocks，sacrum
煎厥	fried-coma
薄厥	oppressed-coma
痤痱	small furuncles，prickly heats
大丁	big malignant boils
祝由	treatment by sorcerer
怒则气上	anger makes the *qi* ascending

喜则气缓	joy makes the *qi* slack
悲则气消	sorrow makes the *qi* depleted
恐则气下	fear makes the *qi* descending
寒则气收	cold makes the *qi* astringent
热则气泄	heat makes the *qi* discharged
惊则气乱	fright makes the *qi* chaotic
劳则气耗	labor makes the *qi* exhausted
思则气结	thought makes the *qi* bound
辩证	syndrome identification
论治	treatment determination
正气	right *qi*
邪气	evils
募原	wrapping membranes of the intestines and stomach
缓筋	sinews of the stomach
脊筋	paravertebral sinews
风者善行而数变	wind tends to run and changes frequently
痹	impediment（numbness）
周痹	whole-body impediment
众痹	multitude impediment
宗筋	ancestral sinew
独取阳明	exclusively select the bright-*yang*（stomach）
痿	atrophy
厥	*qi* reversal
痰	phlegm
饮	rheum
瘀	stasis
积	accumulation
聚	gathering
痈	*yang* carbuncle
疽	*yin* carbuncle
瘅	hot-organ diseases
消渴	depletion-thirst
癫狂	madness，mania
真脏脉	pulse of genuine *zang*-organ
望	observation
闻	auscultation and olfaction

问	interrogation
切	pulse-feeling and palpation
四诊合参	correlation of the four examinations
弦脉	string-like pulse
钩脉	surging and full pulse (hook-like pulse)
毛脉	floating pulse (feather-like pulse)
石脉	sinking pulse (stone-like pulse)
浮脉	floating pulse
沉脉	sinking pulse
弱脉	weak pulse
结脉	irregularly interrupted pulse
代脉	regularly interrupted pulse
涩脉	uneven pulse
缓脉	moderate pulse
滑脉	slippery pulse
细脉	thready pulse
紧脉	tight pulse
数脉	rapid pulse
洪脉	surging pulse
大脉	large pulse
濡脉	soggy pulse
虚里	vacuous interior
尺肤	cubital skin
下极	lower extreme
寒者热之	cold is treated with heat
热者寒之	heat is treated with cold
微者逆之	the slight is treated straight
甚者从之	the serious is treated paradoxically
坚者削之	hardness is whittled away
客者除之	settling is treated by eliminating
劳者温之	fatigue is treated by warming
结者散之	binding is treated by dissipating
留者攻之	lingering is treated by attacking
燥者濡之	dryness is treated by moistening
急者缓之	spasm is treated by relaxing
散者收之	scattering is treated by astringing

损者温之	weakness is treated by warming
逸者行之	comfort is treated by moving
惊者平之	fright is treated by calming
上之下之	raising and lowering
摩之浴之	massaging and bathing
薄之劫之	eroding and plundering
开之发之	opening and emanating
顺	favorable (obedient)
逆	unfavorable (disobedient)
标	tip
本	root
正治(逆治)	straight treatment
反治(从治)	paradoxical treatment
已病	formed disease
未病	unformed disease
热因热用	treat heat with heat
寒因寒用	treat cold with cold
塞因塞用	treat the obstructed by obstructing
通因通用	treat the free by freeing
君臣佐使	monarch, minister, assistant, envoy

图书在版编目(CIP)数据

黄帝内经:英文/朱明译
—北京:外文出版社,2001.1
ISBN 7 – 119 – 02664 – X

Ⅰ.黄… Ⅱ.朱… Ⅲ.内经 – 英文 Ⅳ.R221

中国版本图书馆 CIP 数据核字(2000) 第 61338 号

责任编辑　胡开敏
英文审订　张明捷
封面设计　唐少文

Website :
http://www.flp.com.cn
Email Address :
Info@flp.com.cn
Sales@flp.com.cn

黄　帝　内　经
朱　明　译
*
ⓒ外文出版社
外文出版社出版
(中国北京百万庄大街 24 号)
邮政编码 100037
北京外文印刷厂印刷
中国国际图书贸易总公司发行
(中国北京车公庄西路 35 号)
北京邮政信箱第 399 号　邮政编码 100044
2001 年(16 开) 第 1 版
2005 年第 1 版第 2 次印刷
(英)
ISBN 7 – 119 – 02664 – X/R·183(外)
09000(精)
7 – E – 3385S